Beyond Buds

Next Generation

Beyond Buds: Next Generation — Marijuana Extracts and Cannabis Infusions
by Ed Rosenthal with Greg Zeman

Copyright © 2018 Ed Rosenthal
Published by Quick American
A Division of Quick Trading Co.
Piedmont, CA, USA

ISBN: 978-1-936807-38-3
eISBN: 978-1-936807-39-0

Printed in the United States
First Printing

Editors and Project Managers: Rolph Blythe, Darcy Thompson
Contributing Editor: Josh Sheets
Art Director: Christian Petke
Design: Scott Idleman / Blink
Cover Design: Christian Petke, D-Core
Photo Editors: Darcy Thompson, Christian Petke

Cover Photography: Anthony Buchanan / Constant Concentrates

Library of Congress Control Number: 2018953794

Beyond Buds

Next Generation

Marijuana Concentrates and Cannabis Infusions

Ed Rosenthal with Greg Zeman

ACKNOWLOWLEDGMENTS

Kristen Angelo, (A Pot Farmer's Daughter), Rolph Blythe, Anthony Buchanan, CaliGold, Arya Campbell, Shalaun Curry, The Dank Duchess, Lizzy Fritz, Kyle Gairhan, Guild Extracts, Harmony Extracts, Julia Hass, Heylo Labs, Ellen Holland, Scott Idleman, Chris Jones, Kind Medicine, Jane Klein, LEVEL, Brandon Mondo (Woko), Olala Labs, The Original Resinator, Mermaid Wisdom, Fred Morlege, Oakland Extracts, Christian Petke, Pissing Excellence, Chris Romaine (Kandid Kush) Ramona Rubin, Sashquash, Josh Sheets, Marisa Sympson, Darcy Thompson, Marisa Timko, Forrest White, Evan X (High Noon SF), Will X (Terp Boys).

High Time

The wheels are muddy, got a ton of hay,
Now listen here, Baby, 'cause I mean what I say,

Nothing's for certain, it could always go wrong
Come in when it's raining, go on out when it's gone
We could have us a high time, living the good life, well I know.

—Jerry Garcia / Robert Hunter
Courtesy of the Grateful Dead

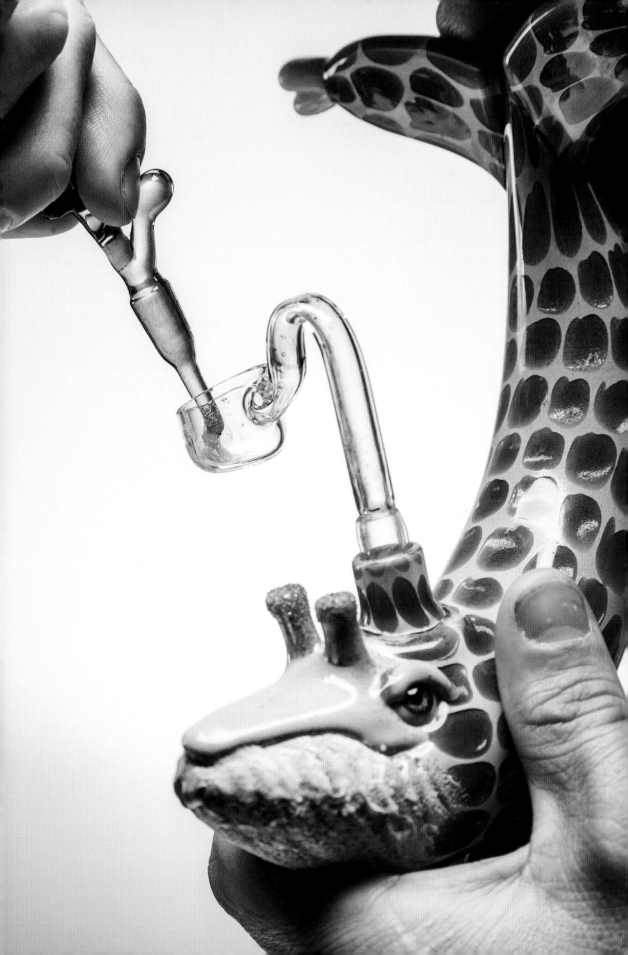

Contents

Part 2: Solvent Based Extraction Methods

Part 3: Solventless Extraction Methods

Part 3: Non-Smokable Methods of Consumption

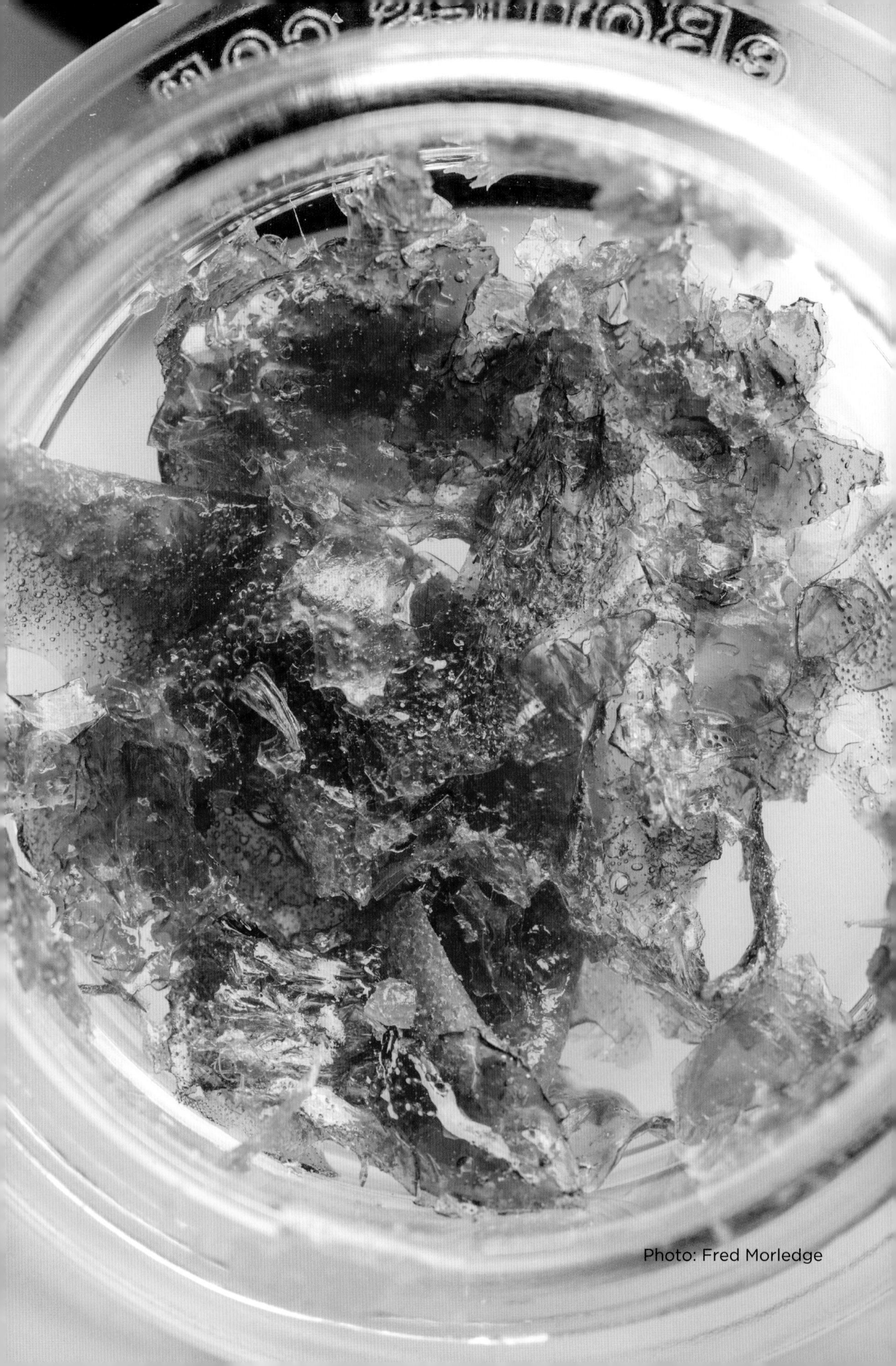

Photo: Fred Morledge

Introduction

By Ellen Holland

Concentrating cannabis, or extracting cannabinoids such as THC and CBD to produce a stronger high, is not a new artform. Cannabis resin in the form of hashish appears in ancient texts. What is new, however, is the advanced extraction methods producers have developed to create "dabbable" extracts. These techniques, explored in depth throughout this book, have resulted in not only the most flavorful, potent smoking experiences, but also in a full paradigm shift for cannabis consumption. The widespread advancements in dabbing have brought concentrates to the "center stage of the commercial and cultural cannabis conversation" and continues to rapidly advance, shooting as fast as a comet straight into the stoner stratosphere.

The two authors of this book, Ed Rosenthal and Greg Zeman, are two of the most knowledgeable cannabis authors of our time. Each brings along years of research, writing and experimentation. But it's their shared highly inquisitive and continually questioning nature geared towards understanding everything about the botanical that makes them unstoppable.

In *Beyond Buds, Next Generation* they join with other passionate marijuana enthusiasts in the desire to experience and explore the purest essence of cannabis. With extracts, the plant material of cannabis is stripped away to distill high concentrations of cannabinoids and terpenes — the aromatic molecules present in cannabis and other plants that can affect moods and physical conditions — resulting in a flavorful hit followed by an immediate high.

As this book explains, there are several different methods for creating cannabis extracts, mostly depending on which type of solvent is used to remove the cannabinoids and terpenes from the plant, and with each comes a whole new set of techniques and terms.

In addition, there are a number of ways to consume cannabis concentrates which, mirroring the ways they are created, are also getting more technical. From vape pens and e-nails to low temp dabs with torches and quartz bangers, there is a advanced set of ways to consume cannabis concentrates and with that comes a brand-new cultural vernacular.

The language, art and science of cannabis concentrates are in full kaleidoscopic display within this book. Enjoy the deep dive into the sea of trichomes and distribute the knowledge with others by learning some of the techniques and sharing the fruits of your own flowers.

Ellen Holland
Senior Editor of *Cannabis Now*

Author's note

By Greg Zeman

A loosely rolled joint of bland Mexican brick weed smoked furtively in the basement garage of a neighbor's house at 2am — this was my introduction to cannabis. Looking back on it now I'm struck by how bad that first joint was compared to last one I smoked, but it was still good enough to spark a lifelong fascination and love affair with one of our planet's most valuable plants.

The way we connect with cannabis has changed dramatically since those days. For a long time the perceived quality of bud was predominantly based on its "potency," which used to be shorthand for how much THC was in it. Cultivation became a THC arms race, with everyone pushing for higher numbers to put on their jar labels. I now laugh when I remember that 13% THC used to be considered so ludicrously strong that there was an urban legend about secret government research bud — the infamous G-13.

Today we have a much better understanding of the physiological impacts of cannabis than ever before. THC is no longer seen as the alpha and omega where effects are concerned. We now know that there are other cannabis compounds like CBD that work in tandem with THC to produce the physical and psychological benefits of cannabis consumption, and that even the organic compounds that create the unique flavors and smells of different strains help to inform the way those strains affect us.

Extraction has pushed the boundaries of our conception of cannabis, forcing us to reconsider what gives the cannabis experience value. Potency is now a given, allowing cultivators to refocus their breeding efforts on selecting more flavorful phenotypes. Terpene profiles are now the dominant indicator of quality, for everything from buds to butter. The new movement in cannabis edibles isn't hiding the flavor of weed, but celebrating it through recipes crafted around its many unique flavor expressions.

We've arranged this book in a way that informs both those new to cannabis and those well versed in dabbing and extraction culture. We begin with a discussion of the cannabis plant's key active compounds — cannabinoids and terpenes — then move on to outline the new ways cannabis is consumed. From there we give readers a tour of next generation extracts, starting with the solvent-based methods; then delve into solventless methods for making dabbable concentrates. Finally, we've provided some new ideas emerging around topical applications, tinctures and edibles, because the new wave of cannabis processing really has changed everything.

A project as ambitious as ours could never be achieved by two people. Thankfully Ed and I had access to some of the brightest minds in cannabis, from chemists, to cultivators, extractors and innovators who generously shared their expertise.

Finally, I'd like to dedicate this book to the memory of my mother, Susan Zeman, who found immense joy and relief in cannabis and whose vibrant curiosity about all things set me on a path of exploration.

A lot of love, dedication and dabs went into making this book a reality; it's my sincere hope that you'll have as much fun reading it as we had writing it.

—Greg Zeman

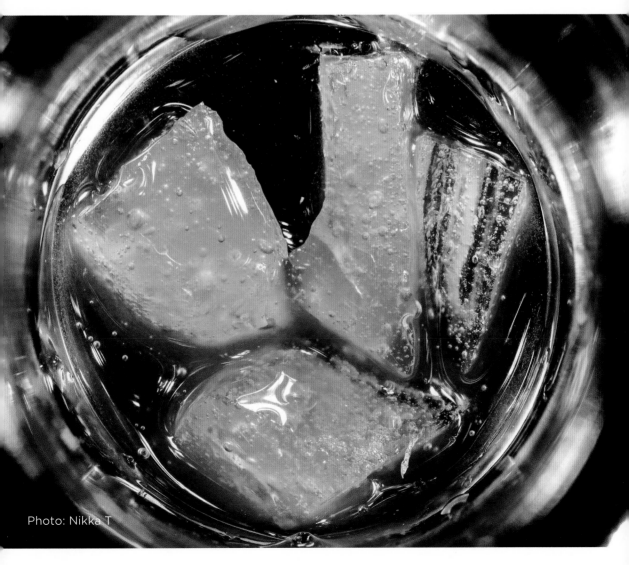

Photo: Nikka T

Photo: Professor P / Dynasty Genetics

CHAPTER 1

Terpenes & Cannabinoids

When the Chinese philosopher Lao-tzu composed the *Tao Te Ching*, one of the foundational texts of Taoism, he wrote the now famous line "a journey of a thousand miles begins with a single step." Where the cannabis plant is concerned, that first step is always a single seed: Every cannabis cultivar's journey begins in a tiny craft that whisks its genetic identity through time, space, and soil into the light of existence.

Where the cannabis *experience* is concerned THC was previously assumed to be the singular "seed" of the plant's famous effects. That misconception informed the approach taken by most cultivators, instilling in them (and by extension, most cannabis consumers) a myopic focus on "potency" gauged by THC concentration: As far as the general public was concerned, more THC meant "stronger" cannabis. As is generally the case, the truth is a bit less tidy but far more interesting.

We'll be sharing a journey of discovery in this book, and our first step will be to explore the essential building blocks of the cannabis experience — cannabinoids and terpenes. Because these compounds are behind the desirable impacts of cannabis consumption, they are also the key target of extraction, the suite of physical and chemical processes used to separate those active ingredients from the inert plant matter and create concentrates. We'll be covering most of the contemporary extraction methods, but first let's orient ourselves around *what* we're extracting and *why*.

CANNABINOIDS

TETRAHYDROCANNABINOL (THC)

This is the cannabinoid every cannabis consumer has heard of; for decades it was perceived as a solo act — *the* psychoactive compound of cannabis.

In 1964 Dr. Raphael Mechoulam, an organic chemist from Israel, first synthesized the delta-9 THC molecule. Pharmacologists released synthesized THC under the brand-name Marinol® in the early 1980s, but the majority of existing cannabis patients say it doesn't provide the same analgesic and anti-inflammatory effects when compared to whole cannabis medicine. Numerous early patient trials comparing synthetic THC and natural cannabis medicine confirmed this patient preference, including one from the Tennessee Board of Pharmacy, conducted to gauge their comparative efficacy as a remedy for vomiting or nausea from chemotherapy. The study found a 23% higher "success rate" for chemo patients who smoked natural cannabis versus those who ingested synthetic THC capsules.[1]

A similar early patient trial conducted at the University of New Mexico[2] found an even more dramatic difference in efficacy, deeming inhalation "far superior" to ingestion — over 90% of patients using inhaled cannabis experienced improvement in their condition, versus just under 60% who improved using oral ingestion.

These same general findings are echoed by other early studies from New York, California, and elsewhere, with more recent research into cannabis use patterns showing a continued preference for natural cannabis by patients with access to both natural and synthetic treatment options.[3]

Additionally, synthetic THC afflicts many users with pronounced side effects not experienced with natural cannabis medicine. Clinical data[4] point to a synergistic relationship between cannabinoids other than THC, as well as the input of terpenes on the entourage effect. Cannabis researchers have found that, not only do terpenes, flavonoids, and other non-THC cannabinoids seem to boost anti-inflammatory effects, stimulate cortical activity, and augment blood flow to the brain, they also "may reduce THC-induced anxiety, cholinergic deficits, and immunosuppression."[5]

While more double-blind studies and clinical research still needs to be done to further verify the scientific validity of the entourage effect, there is a deep catalog of established science on the matter, much of it pointing to real benefits from the combination of multiple cannabinoids and terpenes.

While there's no doubt that THC no longer enjoys solitary celebrity status, it's still a star player in the cannabis experience. If anything, high levels of THC are expected in buds or concentrates sold today, so it isn't as if consumers have lost their "taste" for THC, they've simply expanded their palate to include other offerings.

For a more detailed rundown of how to maximize the THC content of your buds, refer to my book *Marijuana Harvest: Maximizing Quality and Yield in Your Cannabis Garden*. The main trick is to select potent strains with high resin output and time your harvest based on the appearance of the resin glands — clear or milky, not yellow or amber, which indicates a late harvest and (usually) an undesirable concentration of cannabinol or CBN.

CBD

CBD was isolated in the early 1930s, but its structure was not discovered until 1963. Dr. Mechoulam actually synthesized CBD a year before his work with THC. In fact, he isolated THC *from* CBD isolate. But despite that, CBD is still the new kid on the block when it comes to popular cannabis medicine. Once a little known member of THC's entourage, CBD now commands a massive presence, inspiring CBD only decriminalization bills, as well as a booming retail industry of CBD-only products.

Although CBD is often referred to in popular media and marketing materials as "nonpsychoactive," this is a bit of a misnomer. While it's true that CBD is more or less non-intoxicating and will not get you "high" in the same way THC does, it crosses the blood-brain barrier and has some pronounced pharmacological impacts on anxiety, addiction and other mental illnesses, including schizophrenia and depression.

[1] Board of Pharmacy, State of Tennessee. 1983. Annual Report: Evaluation of Marijuana and Tetrahydrocannabinol in Treatment of Nausea and/or Vomiting Associated with Cancer Therapy Unresponsive to Conventional Anti-Emetic Therapy: Efficacy and Toxicity. p. 5.
[2] Behavioral Health Services Division. 1983. The Lynn Pierson Therapeutic Research Program: A Report on Progress to Date. Health and Environment Department: New Mexico. p. 4.
[3] D. Prentiss et al. 2004. Patterns of marijuana use among patients with HIV/AIDS followed in a public health care setting. *Journal of Acquired Immune Deficiency Syndromes* 35: 38–45.
[4] E. Williamson. 2001. Synergy and other interactions in phytomedicines. Phytomedicine: *International Journal of Phytotherapy and Phytopharmacology* 8: 401–409.
[5] J. McPartland and E. Russo. 2002. Cannabis and cannabis extracts: greater than the sum of their parts. *Journal of Cannabis Therapeutics*. p. 103.

BENEFITS OF CBD ISOLATE

Interest in CBD is growing because of its incredible health benefits. Its anti-inflammatory, anti-spasmodic, and anti-anxiety properties are just a sampling of the attributes researchers have unearthed, and manufacturers have tapped into. Patients suffering from diseases as varied as Alzheimer's and multiple sclerosis have reported experiencing relief after consuming CBD.

CBD also doesn't have any intoxicating effects. A pure CBD isolate will affect your body, but your mind will remain clear. The "high" feeling that THC creates is highly sought after by many consumers, but others are mainly interested in the other potential health benefits. In fact, CBD has been shown to counterbalance the intoxicating effects of THC.

Isolating specific cannabinoids has become a huge part of the cannabis industry. Currently, interest is primarily focused on THC and CBD, but that is evolving as legalization sweeps the country and research dollars pour into the industry.

There is significant scientific rationale for mixing CBD and THC together to produce increased pleasurable effects: A study that co-administered the two cannabinoids found that "CBD also changed the symptoms in such a way that the subjects receiving the mixtures showed less anxiety and panic but reported more pleasurable effects."

TETRAHYDROCANNABINOLIC ACID (THCa) & CANNABIDIOLIC ACID (CBDa)

Many people don't realize that even "high THC" cultivars of the cannabis plant produce very little psychoactive delta-9-THC; the vast majority of what's contained inside the resin glands is THCa, the chemical precursor of THC. The same is true for CBD: High CBD strains are actually high in CBDa. In both instances, the "a" stands for acid — carboxylic acid specifically, which does not easily pass through the blood-brain barrier because of its atomic structure, which is altered passively through the process of decarboxylation; the name refers to the removal of the COOH "carboxyl group."

Throughout this book, we'll discuss various processes for extracting cannabinoid acids without decarboxylating them. Although people generally refer to the total measured potency of a flower or concentrate (including acidic precursors) as "cannabinoid content," it's the raw cannabinoid acids that are dominant in bud. Smoking, vaporizing, or in some caeses extracting the bud decarboxylates THCA to delta-9-THC, the psychoactive compound, or in the case of cannabidiol (CBD), from CBDa to CBD. There are several extraction and post-extraction methods for decarboxylating different products, which all rely on the application of heat and are covered in the respective chapters for those products.

The transformation of cannabinoid acids to psychoactive cannabinoids also occurs over time without the addition of heat through oxidation that occurs during the natural drying and curing process. It's important to keep in mind that any process that converts THCa to THC also converts some THC to CBN.

There are many uses for the raw, acidic form of cannabinoids; many tinctures utilize them because they offer several of the same benefits of the decarboxylated form, but with reduced intoxication. While tincture techniques are covered in their dedicated chapter it's important to understand the difference between raw and "activated" cannabinoids, because they have different properties and impacts: many patients find great relief in combining both.

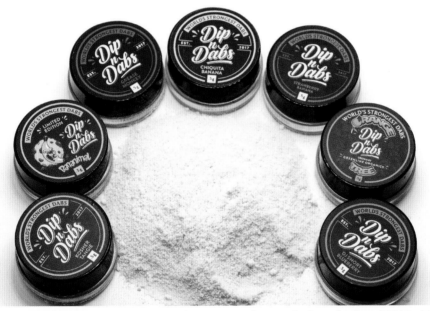

Pacific Organic and Wellness' Dip n Dabs are powder made from isolated THCa. The containers are strain-specific and re-introduce the plant's terpenes to maintain the flavor, aroma and effect profile of the original flower strains.

WHAT IS THCA ISOLATE?

Isolating THCa means isolating the active ingredient in cannabis before it is activated. When ingested, THCa is nonpsychoactive but has medicinal properties such as anti-inflammation, anti-nausea, and pain relief. When dabbed or smoked, the THC activates, delivering a powerful, energetic high with very little body sedation. This makes THCa a unique cannabinoid because you can eat or drink it without getting "high," or you can smoke it to release higher levels of THC. Strain specific THCa, from brands like Dip 'n' Dabs are strain specific. The company has reintroduce the same strain's terpenes to maintain the original flavor, aroma, and effect profile..

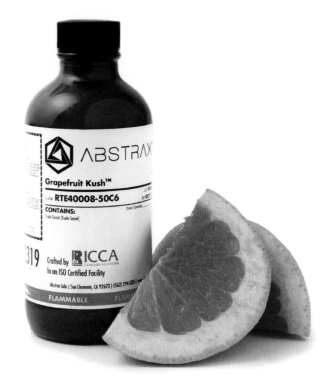

Many extraction methods strip the plant of natural, flavorful terpenes, causing companies to add plant-based terpenes back into their products.. Ricca's Abstrax line includes terpene blends like Grapefruit Kush hybrid, a crossbreed of the grapefruit and BC Kush strains.

The cold extraction processes discussed in this book preserve the raw, acidic cannabinoids. Extraction methods that use high enough temperatures produce decarboxylated, neutral (versus acidic) cannabinoids.

A simple example is the difference between bud and brownies: If you take an eighth of high-potency bud and eat it, there will be little-to-no noticeable effects. That doesn't mean there won't be any benefits — many people swear by juicing and consuming raw cannabis for improved health and wellness — but it certainly won't get you high. This is because the vast majority of the cannabinoids in the bud have not been decarboxylated, so they remain in their raw, non-intoxicating state.

A brownie, on the other hand, has been exposed to temperatures exceeding THC's decarb point, which is right around 220°F. Even if you didn't decarb your bud before making butter and baking, it is possible you still baked at a temp higher than the decarb point, so the vast majority of the cannabinoids in your brownie are active THC, meaning if you eat it, well, you know what happens. This same rule applies to CBD, only the decarb point is slightly higher — roughly 280°F.

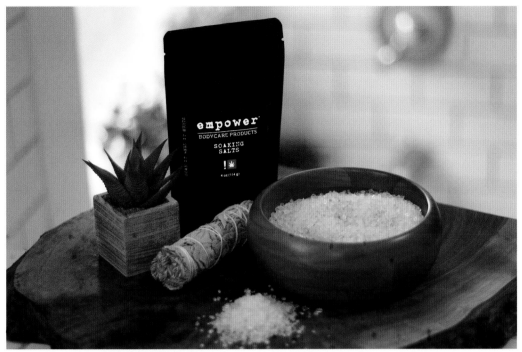

Empower® Soaking Salts are infused with THCa, CBD and THC. Combining even a small amount of THC with CBD has been shown to assist the uptake of CBD and thereby increase the health benefits.

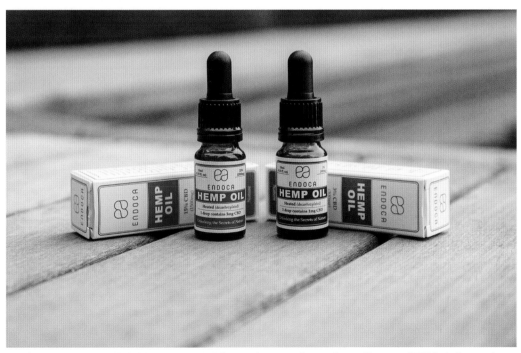

Endoca's Hemp Oil delivers CBD without the psychoactive effects of THC. It is made from hemp seeds rich in Omegas 3 and 6.

THE ENTOURAGE EFFECT

In 1998, Dr. Mechoulam and his team introduced the idea of the entourage effect. This research validated the hypothesis that different cannabinoids work synergistically on the endo-cannabinoid system, enhancing their activity. When smoked on its own, CBD has been shown to have positive physiological effectson the body. These include parasympathetic nervous system activation and appetite induction. Combined with THC, it reduces the paranoia and anxiety normally associated with cannabis use.

Some of the seminal scientific studies on this effect were done in Brazil in the 1970's. Studying the habits of recreational users and the effects of chronic use, re-searchers found that high doses of THC on its own produced anxiety and panic—but adding CBD significantly reduced those symptoms in patients. The subjects receiving the mixtures showed less anxiety and panic but reported more pleasurable effects.

Pharmacologically, there is a host of evidence mixing THC and CBD together is beneficial. Sativex®, made by GW Pharmaceuticals, is one of only two cannabis-derived prescription medications available for use. Containing a 1:1 mixture of THC:CBD, as well as trace amounts of other cannabinoids from the whole-cannabis extraction process, Sativex® has been shown to treat multiple sclerosis (MS) and to reduce the pain-reduction threshold in terminal cancer patients.

More studies are needed to show how our favorite cannabinoid cousins can best pair together to create the desired effects.

CBD FOR ANXIETY

One unique study discussed the effects of CBD on social anxiety in people and the underlying neural processes associated with it. Patients were either given an oral dose of CBD or a placebo. The study focused illustrated that CBD indeed reduced social anxiety.

As cannabis becomes legalized in more states, additional studies will bolster the existing research showing that CBD can remove the anxiety, physical response, and fear of illnesses like PTSD.

Lulu's CBD Chocolates contain wild-harvested, fair trade, heirloom, unroasted cacao beans. They produce an 80mg CBD : zero THC bar, or a 20mg CBD single serving.

MIDNIGHT VELVET

CBD FOR SLEEP

CBD has powerful anxiolytic effects that improves sleep biomarkers (including onset) helping sleep patterns reset. According to a Brazilian case study, the administration of CBD was associated with significantly decreased anxiety and increased mental sedation. So, if anxiety and stress is the cause of sleeping issues, CBD can help break that cycle, allowing for more natural sleep patterns.

Another study suggests that CBD attaches to the endocannabinoid receptors CB1 and CB2 within the body which work in tandem to maintain homeostasis. It found that arthritis sufferers have a higher concentration of C2 receptors in their joints, and when CBD interacted with those receptors, promoting analgesia in the affected area.

CBD also allows those who wake up in the middle of the night to stay asleep. One study showed that CBD can improve complex sleep-related behaviors associated with rapid eye movement (REM). Another found that CBD's anxiolytic effects were responsible for blocking REM sleep suppression typical of PTSD symptoms.

Five to ten milligrams of CBD per day is a good starting dose. If your main problem is anxiety or pain, take a CBD tincture sublingually or through a gel capsule, one or two hours before bed. For those who wake up in the middle of the night, use a vaporizer when it occurs for instant effects to help you fall back asleep. If you feel this dosage is not enough, gradually increase it by 5-10 milligram increments until the desired effect is achieved.

Thanks to the research on CBD, many people are benefitting from this wonderful non-psychoactive cannabinoid. Just remember, there is no universal method of using CBD, it all depends on what results you are trying to achieve.

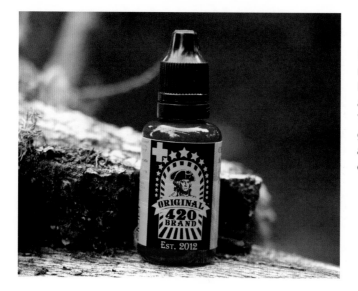

Many CBD tinctures are made from hemp oil. Others like the Original 420 Brand are made from a CBD isolate. With an organic vegetable glycerin base and strawberry and white-peach flavors. It comes in various strengths.

CBN

As mentioned previously, CBN has long been considered undesirable in high concentration by most cannabis consumers and, by extension, cultivators. This is because CBN is produced through the degradation of THC through exposure to oxygen (oxidization) and THC has traditionally been the most desirable cannabinoid. CBN levels rise naturally as mature cannabis plants near harvest, because the same oxidation process that converts THCa to THC also transforms THC to CBN.

CBN levels also increase during decarboxylation; exposure to heat increases the natural degradation process, meaning THCa is being converted to delta-9-THC, which is simultaneously being converted to CBN. That balancing act has long been biased towards maximizing delta-9 levels and minimizing CBN concentration, but as the way the public consumes and relates to cannabis evolves to encompass more cannabinoids there is a small but growing interest in CBN extracts.

Traditionally, most cannabis consumer experiences with CBN have come from consuming old buds that have converted most of their THC to CBN through gradual oxidation. This experience is generally characterized by the effect most associated with CBN — somnolence, or sleep induction. Those seeking the effects they enjoyed a year ago (never mind the long since volatized terpene profile) will be disappointed, but those just trying to get a good night's sleep might appreciate the extra CBN.

As with all cannabinoids, CBN can be isolated through fractional distillation for use in tinctures or consumption through dabbing, but there are very few commercial sources for these products at present. This could represent an opportunity moving forward as demand for cannabinoids beyond THC and CBD gradually expands with our understanding of their respective contribution to the entourage effect and their individual impacts.

CBGA: THE MOTHER OF ALL CANNABINOIDS

If you've never heard of cannabigerol or CBG you aren't alone — many cannabis consumers are unaware of this "minor" cannabinoid, which generally only appears in minute concentration (1% or less) in harvested cannabis. However, without this precursor cannabinoid there would be no THC or CBD.

All THCa and CBDa contained in the resin glands of the cannabis plant starts out as CBGa, which is internally produced and subsequently converted by enzymes into THCa, CBDa or CBCa — another cannabinoid which is just appearing on the radars of researchers in earnest.

But, as with all cannabinoids, we're learning that CBG has its own distinct impacts on human physiology, which include inhibiting cancer cell growth and reducing intraocular pressure.

CBC

Cannabichromene is "nonpsychoactive," in the sense that it doesn't bind readily to CB1 cannabinoid receptors. It does seem to provide analgesic effects though, and has been shown to bond with pain receptors. Research into this cannabinoid is still thin compared to the voluminous data on CBD and THC, but it has been show to have a unique affect on anandamide, an endocannabinoid associated with numerous therapeutic effects, from alleviating depression to inhibiting cancer cell growth. CBC allows anandamide to remain in the bloodstream for longer, increasing its cumu-lative impact and boosting its efficacy. This effect has also been observed with CBD, but early research suggests it may be even more pronounced with CBC.

A NOTE ON THE ENDOGENOUS CANNABINOID SYSTEM (ECS)

Dr. Mechoulam's many contributions to cannabis medicine also include the discovery of the human body's natural cannabis receptor system. This physiological system is responsible for maintaining homeostasis throughout the body at a cellular level.

One important task that exemplifies the broad stabilizing power of the endogenous cannabinoid system (ECS) is the way it responds to physical injury; at the site of the trauma, you will find cannabinoids handling three specific biological mechanisms simultaneously:

- Suppressing the release of sensitizers and activators
- Stabilizing nerve cells to reduce firing
- Inhibiting the release of inflammatory agents into nearby immune cells

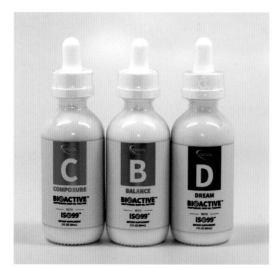

This Bioactive Adaptogenic Hemp Oil ™ from Isodiol is available as a tincture. The products are used to promote mental clarity, relaxation and restful sleep.

All three of these "tasks" handled by the ECS serve the same function: reducing pain at the site of the injury. This same biological balancing act takes place at every level of the body all the time; the ECS is always working to maintain homeostasis.

Cannabinoids don't just feel good because your body *likes* them; they're fundamental components of human health.

We won't delve too deeply into the ECS. However, for those looking to gain a fuller understanding of the ways the products outlined in this book impact the human body, there are resources for further reading in the suggested texts at the end.

UNPACKING "MORE RESEARCH IS NEEDED"

It's like clockwork. Any discussion on cannabis medicine and the science behind how cannabis works inevitably ends up with somebody saying that phrase — the last rhetorical sanctuary of the status quo on cannabis — "more research is needed."

And of course there is some truth to that. Any social and scientific phenomenon with as many facets and developing fronts as cannabis undoubtedly requires a monumental undertaking by researchers and scientists to better understand it. However, this ignores the mountain of very legitimate clinical research already logged on this topic, much of it originating in Israel, which has a less restrictive legal environment when it comes to cannabis research.

It is our sincere hope that research into cannabis continues forever, but we also can't let advocates of prohibition conflate the endless need for more knowledge with an absence of sufficient data to move forward with decriminalization.

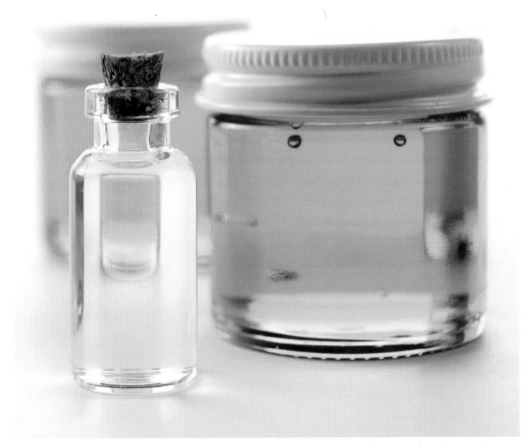

Wildseed Oil is an example of a socially-conscious cannabis brand focused on undoing some of the harms caused by the drug war. The company donates 20% of their profits to applicable organizations. Their website contains links to articles and studies that provide answers to claims that "more research is needed."

TERPENES

Terpenes are the primary organic building blocks of the essential oils. These oils produce the odors we associate with plants, especially the flowers and fruit.

Together, cannabis varieties offer a diverse representation of the natural terpene spectrum. Depending on genetics — and the phenotypical expression of those genes — a cannabis flower can express a myriad of odors, including flowers, fruits, vegetables as well as skunk, leather, baked goods and chemical odors like gasoline and diesel.

This chapter will delve into the numerous ways terpenes in-fluence the cannabis experience, but let's not overlook the core function of terpenes — they make cannabis taste and smell incredible. We're learning so much about the ways terpenes inform the effects of consumption, but that's only happening because cannabis culture has shifted from a myopic focus on THC towards nuanced appreciation of unique "flavor profiles."

The new renaissance in cannabis extraction has both driven and responded to this shift: The next generation of extraction allows for isolation of these flavor profiles, delivering a clear expression of the terps without interference from waxes, chlorophyll and other inert compounds present in the cannabis plant. Since high potency is a given with concentrates, less focus is put on potency during cultivation, allowing cultivators and breeders to focus on developing flavorful phenotypes. But terpenes do much more than taste and smell delicious: Terps don't just make Trainwreck *smell* different than OG Kush, they're also responsible for the radically different ways those varieties make you feel. So as breeders produce new, novel terpene profiles consumers are also enjoying unique suites of effects.

The entourage effect illustrates the way CBD, other cannabinoids and terpenes work in concert with THC to produce the varied effects of cannabis. Terpenes imbue cannabis flowers with their prismatic range of aromas and help create the characteristic effects of a given strain. Essential oils contain terpenes and their impact on mind, brain and body have been the focus of aromatherapy. Think of cannabis consumption as enhanced aromatherapy. The effects of terpenes are amplified by cannabinoids, the ratio of which also dictates the way your body chemistry interacts with a dose of cannabis.

TEREPENE EFFECTS AND AROMATHERAPY

The word "aromatherapy" was never used until the early 1900s, when the practice experienced a renaissance and subsequent rebranding, but it has roots in the ancient world, which highly prized fragrant gums, oils and resins for their perceived meditative and medicinal properties. So the idea of using the body's olfactory system as a delivery system for medicine is nothing new, but as with the equally ancient practice of herbal medicine, our understanding of the verifiable science behind why it does (or sometimes doesn't) work is still under construction.

The scientific understanding of *how* terpenes affect the human body is still developing, but what is known for certain is that — irrespective of the precise physiological mechanism and pathway — there is some measurable impact from exposure to and/or ingestion of terpenes. This disconnect between our observation of the aromatherapy phenomenon and our understanding of it is summed up neatly by a 2013 study that attempted to quantify the therapeutic impacts of limonene on mice using standardized methodology:

"Many essential oils have relaxing properties and have long been used traditionally in folk medicine (Lawless, 2002). However, few studies have been conducted using standardized methodology to demonstrate the anxiolytic-like effects of these fragrances when administered by inhalation, as in aromatherapy... These data indicate that (+)-limonene can be used as an anti-anxiety agent in aromatherapy. Nonetheless, further studies should be conducted to clarify the mechanism of its anxiolytic-like effects."

So we know that terpenes really do directly impact human physiology, and while we don't know exactly how they do it that hasn't stopped other industries from embracing their power.

One example of the psychological effect terpenes can have is the commercial application of aromatherapy through "ambient scent branding" or "aroma branding" to influence consumer behavior. Merchants have been using this general principle for generations — at least since ancient Chinese merchants perfumed their silks to boost sales. The contemporary expression of aroma branding — which involves diffusing specially formulated scents through air conditioning systems — was largely pioneered by the hospitality industry in the early '90s.

One of the first hotels to install such a system was the Mirage Hotel and Casino in Las Vegas, Nevada in 1991. These systems rapidly evolved from smoke odor control solutions to what is now perceived as a powerful tool for influencing guest behavior and establishing brand identity; a 2009 study postulated the now prevailing belief that certain scents can reduce risk aversion in gamblers, resulting in longer playtime. There have been criticisms of the study's methodology, but almost every major Vegas strip casino hotel now has a "signature" scent that is dispersed throughout the property, in addition to other aromas intended to inspire specific behaviors.

While there are some disagreements over why (or to what extent) the balance of the research on the topic suggests that proper application of aroma branding has a pronounced impact on some areas of consumer behavior. A 2016 study examined and critiqued the previous studies around this practice (including the famous "casino studies" from the 1990s) and performed its own experiment. Their conclusion doesn't pin down a precise mechanism, but it "generally confirm(s) the larger literature from the fields of marketing and psychology which indicates that scents may induce consumers in spending more by increasing their valuation for the product."

Terpenes are powerful compounds with measurable therapeutic effects, which is why they are the primary target of extraction along with cannabinoids.

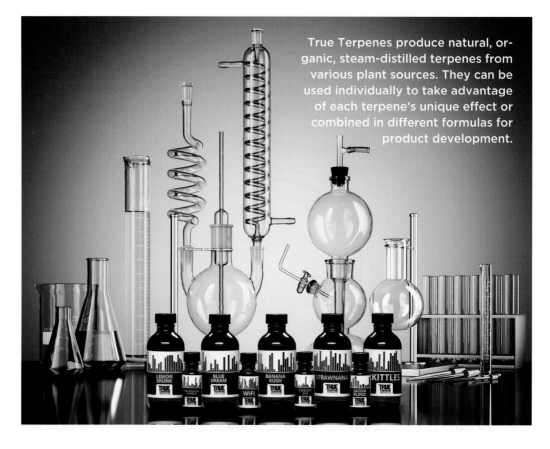

True Terpenes produce natural, organic, steam-distilled terpenes from various plant sources. They can be used individually to take advantage of each terpene's unique effect or combined in different formulas for product development.

A WORD ON TERPENES AND "INDICA OR SATIVA" EFFECTS

So we know that terpene consumption has real physiological effects, and when it comes to cannabis, terpenes are the cornerstone of our new understanding where the respective effects of distinct cultivars/strains is concerned.

While scientific and medical research on the impacts of terpenes in cannabis is still fairly nascent, general information already available about terpenes allows cannabis consumers to make more informed decisions about which flower varieties and products are most likely to provide desired effects.

There was a time not long ago when the primary tool for selecting an appropriate product for treating a given condition or achieving a particular sensation was a crude taxonomy that separated strains into two columns; indica and sativa. Anyone who's been in a cannabis dispensary in the last ten years has heard a similar spiel: Indica provides a heavier "body high" with roughly sedative effects and is best for the evening; Sativa has a stimulating "head high" that offers cerebral impacts with less pronounced physical effects, making it ideal for daytime use. Our new understanding undermines this old "sativa vs. indica" paradigm, but many cannabis consumers discovered the deficiencies in this approach through personal experience, whether that meant smoking a sativa that inspired "couch lock" or an indica that kept them awake all night.

In reality, the distinction of *Cannabis sativa* and *Cannabis indica* is all about the physical characteristics of the plant: sativas tend to grow tall, with lanky structure and slender fan leaves, while indicas are generally shorter, more "squat" in their structure and have broader fan leaves. But none of those physical characteristics have any actual bearing on the chemical impacts of the plant — that all boils down to terpenes and cannabinoids. Additionally, there are very few genetically "pure" indicas or sativas, given the extensive crossbreeding involved in contemporary cannabis cultivation, further complicating the attribution of indica or sativa "effects."

What really determines the impacts of a given variety is how the cannabinoid concentration and ratio interplays with the terpene profile, and here we do find *some* loose correlation between certain terpene profiles associated with indica and sativa effects and actual indica or sativa genetic dominance: Our working hypothesis is that the high levels of myrcene found in many indica strains likely contributes to that suite of effects, and that likewise high levels of limonene, α-pinene and betacarophylene found in sativa dominant strains *may* account for those famous sativa effects.

It isn't difficult to find evidence of this; think of a strain that's considered especially stimulating. You probably thought of something like Trainwreck, Sour Diesel, Tangie, Durban Poison, maybe even Red Congolese. Add a few more of your favorites to that list — see any pattern emerging? Chances are you're seeing certain terpenes repeated across most of those varieties, namely limonene and pinene. This may be another example of "anecdotal data," but when you start exploring the terpene profiles of strains with similar effects you do often find striking similarities.

A WORD ON "ADDED TERPS"

You may have encountered products that claim to "re-add" terpenes lost during extraction. This is often a claim made by extractors of "clear distillate," which uses short path distillation, a process that removes all terpenes. The truth is, while there are undoubtedly some extractors who actually do this, there is little benefit because cannabis-derived terpenes are not especially stable or reliable. Most cannabis terpene profiles in distillate products — the ones that claim to be "OG" or "GG#4" — do not use terpenes actually extracted from those plants. The source material for the *cannabinoid* content may have been the listed cannabis variety, but the added terpene profile is almost certainly a synthetic blend created with food grade terpenes, which are more reliable and stable. There is disagreement about what benefit there may be in preserving natural terpene profiles, but from a chemical standpoint there is no measurable difference between "pure" d-Limonene extracted from cannabis or d-Limonene from orange peels or some other source. For more information on specific qualities associated with terpenes see appendix. For more information on extracting terpenes see the chart that follows and the Fractional & Short Path Distillation chapter in this book.

THE JOURNEY BEGINS . . .

Consuming raw buds will never go completely out of style: Even in the face of our evolving understanding of what specific compounds contribute to the physiological impacts of the plant, there's something viscerally alluring about interacting with it directly. So as methods for extracting the key ingredients behind its desirable effects evolve and improve, so too does the technology around vaporization, which allows for selective consumption of desirable compounds directly off the buds. But concentrates are undoubtedly the new frontier in cannabis — their massive and still-growing popularity is undeniable. The next chapter will break down the ways cannabis consumption has changed in the face of new knowledge and products, which have radically altered the landscape of cannabis culture, and which we'll soon be learning to make.

THE FUTURE OF CANNABIS MEDICINE?

Different strains of cannabis have very different effects. For example, Blue Dream and Sour Diesel both have roughly the same average amount of THC, but they also contain hundreds of different molecules, beyond THC or CBD, that make up the strain. Traditionally, manufacturers use heat to activate and infuse cannabis, but in doing so, they degraded or destroyed the hundreds of molecules that give each strain its unique effects.

What if there was a way to activate cannabinoids while maintaining all of those plant-based molecules? Harvest Direct Enterprises, an innovative biotechnology firm out of Seattle, Washington, is working to address this problem with their proprietary, patent-pending technology: LACY (Lossless Activation Chamber Y).

Lossless activation and infusion of cannabinoids enables manufacturers to more easily put cannabis in forms that doctors and pharmacists are comfortable prescribing and dispensing—such as capsules, inhalers and topicals. The cannabinoid and terpene profiles preserved via LACY can then be used to treat a long list of diseases and ailments related to the endocannabinoid system, including: nausea and vomiting, wasting syndrome (AIDS), lack of appetite (exhibited in cancer and AIDs patients as well as patients suffering from anorexia nervosa), multiple sclerosis, spinal cord trauma, epilepsy, chronic pain, arthritis (and other musculoskeletal disorders), movement disorders, glaucoma, asthma, hypertension, psychiatric disorders, Alzheimer's and dementia, general inflammation, gastrointestinal disorders, and many more.

The ultimate goal is to replace many of the pharmaceutical drugs in our medicine cabinet with a safe, natural, and holistic alternative. This is the future of cannabis medicine.

Diamond
Photo: Professor P / Dynasty Genetics

TERPENE CHART

THE WOODS & THE EARTH

+ FOUND IN **〰 AROMA** **🌡 BOILING POINTS**
♻ MEDICAL PROPERTIES **✳ CANNABIS VARIETIES**

α-Pinene
+ Pine, Rosemary, Parsley
〰 Turpentine, Pine, Dill
🌡 311°F, 155°C
♻ bronchodilator, asthma, anti-inflammatory, aids memory
✳ Jack Herer, Blue Dream, AK-47, Romulan, Harlequin, Kush Group, Cloudburst

Terpinolene
+ Pine, Conifers, Nutmeg, Lilacs
〰 Woods, Smoke, Herbal
🌡 343-347, 361°F, 173-175, 183°C
♻ anti-oxidant, anti-cancer, sedative
✳ Jack Herer, Pineapple Jack, Afghani, Pineapple Kush, OG Group, Durban Poison, XJ-13

Terpineol
+ Pine, Lapsang Souchong tea
〰 Lilac
🌡 426°F, 219°C
♻ anti-oxidant, sedative, anti-inflammatory, anti-malarial, anti-anxiety
✳ Jack Herer, White Widow, Girl Scout Cookies, OG Group, Black Mamba, Skywalker, Blue Cheese

Carene
+ Pine, Cedar
〰 Sweet, Pungent, Woods
🌡 340°F, 171°C
♻ dry out excess bodily fluids (tears, mucus); central nervous system depressant, memory retention, anti-inflammatory
✳ Super Lemon Haze, Skunk #1, Jack Herer, Blueberry Muffin, Trainwreck, XJ-13

Camphene
+ Trees, Citronella, Ginger
〰 Pungent, Musky, Earthy
🌡 318°F, 159°C
♻ pain relief, anti-oxidant
✳ Strawberry Banana, OG Group, Black Mamba, Skywalker, Kush Group, ACDC, Girl Scout Cookies, Truffula Tree

Camphor
+ Camphor tree, Rosemary
〰 Pungent
🌡 408°F, 209°C
♻ readily absorbed through skin, produces cooling sensation like menthol, slight local anesthetic, anti-microbial substance
✳ Black Mamba, Skywalker

Cedrene
+ Cedar
〰 Woods, Cedar
🌡 503°F, 262°C
♻ anti-microbial, anti-fungal, anti-cancer

Guaiol
+ Guaiacum/Cypress trees
〰 Woods, Pine, Rose
🌡 198°F, 92°C
♻ antimicrobial, anti-inflammatory
✳ Chocolope, White Widow, Harlequin, Kush Group, Medical Mass, Dream Queen

Phellandrene
+ Eucalyptus
〰 Mint, Citrus, Pepper
🌡 341°F, 171°C
♻ anti-depressant, anti-cancer, expectorant
✳ Jack Herer, Trainwreck, Arjan's Haze #3, Arjan's Strawberry Haze, XJ-13

Eucalyptol
+ Eucalyptus, Bay Leaves, Tea Tree, Wormwood, Basil
〰 Mint, Earthy, Cool
🌡 349°F, 176°C
♻ anti-fungal, Alzheimer's, anti-inflammatory, asthma, anti-bacterial
✳ Super Silver Haze, Headband, ACDC

PEPPERS & SPICE

+ FOUND IN **〰 AROMA**
🌡 BOILING POINTS **♻ MEDICAL PROPERTIES**
✳ CANNABIS VARIETIES

β-Caryophyllene
+ Black Pepper, Clove, Cinnamon
〰 Peppery, Spicy, Earthy
🌡 260°F, 130°C
♻ epilepsy, anti-anxiety, chronic pain, muscle spasms, insomnia
✳ Girl Scout Cookies, White Widow, Super Silver Haze, Black Mamba, Skywalker, Pineapple Express, Kush Group, Hash Plant, AK47, XJ-13

CITRUS

+ FOUND IN **〰 AROMA**
🌡 BOILING POINTS **♻ MEDICAL PROPERTIES**
✳ CANNABIS VARIETIES

d-Limonene
+ Citrus fruits, Juniper
〰 Citrus
🌡 349°F, 176°C
♻ anti-depressant, GERD, assists with skin absorption of other terpenes
✳ Sour Diesel, Lemon Skunk, Trainwreck, Bubba Kush, OG Group, Black Mamba, Skywalker, AK47

Sabinene
+ Oak, Norway Spruce, Carrot, Nutmeg
〰 Pine, Orange, Spicy
🌡 326°F, 164°C
♻ benefits liver function and digestion, relieves arthritis, and soothe skin conditions
✳ Super Silver Haze, Arjan's Ultra Haze #1

Caryophyllene Oxide
+ Clove, Pepper, Lemon Balm, Lavender, Rosemary
〰 Peppery, Spicy, Earthy
🌡 536°F, 280°C
♻ anti-fungal, anti-coagulant
✳ Durban Poison, XJ-13

Valencene
+ Valencia Oranges
〰 Citrus, Sweet, Herbal, Woods
🌡 253°F, 123°C
♻ anti-inflammatory
✳ Tangie, Agent Orange

Nerolidol
+ Citrus fruits, Jasmine, Tea Tree Oil
〰 Rose, Citrus, Woods
🌡 252°F, 122°C
♻ sedative, potent anti-fungal and anti-malarial activity, anti-oxidant, anti-fungal
✳ Jack Herer, OG Group, Gorilla Glue #4, San Fernando Valley

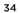

HERBAL

+ FOUND IN   ))) AROMA   🌡 BOILING POINTS
⚕ MEDICAL PROPERTIES   ❈ CANNABIS VARIETIES

Ocimene

+ Mint, Parsley, Basil, Mango
))) Herbal, Sweet, Woods
🌡 212°F, 100°C
⚕ anti-fungal, anti-septic, decongestant, anti-bacterial
❈ Golden Goat, Strawberry Cough, Kush Group, Sour Diesel, Green Crack, Headband

Fenchol

+ Basil
))) Floral, Piney, Woods, Lemony
🌡 394°F, 201°C
⚕ OG Group, Black Mamba, Skywalker, Kush Group, Blue Cheese, Headband, Gelato
❈ Jack Herer, Pineapple Jack, Afghani, Pineapple Kush, OG Group, Durban Poison, XJ-13

Borneol

+ Mugwort, Wormwood, Sagebrush, Tropical Trees, Ginger
))) Herbal, Woods
🌡 415°F, 213°C
⚕ sedative, used for relaxation, anti-inflammatory, anti-nociceptive, anti-coagulant, drug potentiator
❈ Amnesia Haze, Golden Haze, Kush Group, Blue Cheese, OG Group

Bisabolol

+ German Chamomile
))) Tangy, Citrus, Floral, Sweet
🌡 307°F, 153°C
⚕ apoptosis in models of leukemia, anti-inflammatory, anti-bacterial
❈ Harle-Tsu, Headband, ACDC, Oracle, Grape Stomper, Royal Kush, Royal Highness, Blue Cheese, XJ-13

Phytol

+ Green Tea, Green Plants
))) Light Floral, Jasmine, Green Tea
🌡 399°F, 204°C
⚕ inhibits the enzyme that degrades the neurotransmitter GABA, relaxant, prevents Vitamin A teratogenesis, immunosuppressant
❈ Sour Diesel, Cheese, Blue Cheese, Blue Dream, OG Group

Isoborneol

+ Mugwort, Wormwood, Sagebrush, Tropical Trees, Ginger
))) Herbal, Woods
🌡 415°F, 213°C
⚕ antiviral, inhibitor of herpes simplex virus type 1
❈ Amnesia Haze, Golden Haze

Menthol

+ Corn Mint, Peppermint
))) Mint, Menthol
🌡 414°F, 212°C
⚕ analgesic, topical treatment of inflammation
❈ Arjan's Haze #3

Isopulegol

+ Mint
))) Mint, Herbal
🌡 414°F, 212°C
⚕ gastroprotective, anti-inflammatory, reduces seizure severity in animal studies, anti-microbial
❈ Kosher Tangie, Headcheese, Truffula Tree, AMS, Big Bang

Cymene

+ Cumin, Thyme, Coriander, Oregano
))) Orange, Carrot, Turpentine
🌡 351°F, 177°C
⚕ anti-inflammatory, prevents acute lung injury, anti-biotic
❈ Purple Panty Dropper, Jack Herer, Mango Sherbert, Don Carlos

Pulegone

+ Catnip, Mint, Pennyroyal
))) Mint, Camphor
🌡 430°F, 221°C
⚕ acetylcholinesterase inhibitor, aids memory
❈ OG Kush, Headband

FLORAL

+ FOUND IN   ))) AROMA
🌡 BOILING POINTS   ⚕ MEDICAL PROPERTIES
❈ CANNABIS VARIETIES

Linalool

+ Lavender, Bergamot
))) Floral
🌡 388°F, 198°C
⚕ anti-anxiety, sedative, anti-convulsant, pain relief, anti-depressant
❈ Lavender, Headband, Amnesia Haze, LA Confidential, OG Group, Tangerine Dream, AK47

HOPPY

+ FOUND IN   ))) AROMA
🌡 BOILING POINTS   ⚕ MEDICAL PROPERTIES
❈ CANNABIS VARIETIES

Myrcene

+ Hops, Mango, Lemongrass
))) Hoppy, Herbal, Earthy
🌡 333°F, 167°C
⚕ antiseptic, sedative, anti-bacterial, anti-fungal, anti-inflammatory
❈ Blue Dream, Grand Daddy Purple, Northern Lights, Amnesia, Kush Group, Chemdawg

Geraniol

+ Rose, Geraniums, Tobacco
))) Floral
🌡 447°F, 231°C
⚕ anti-oxidant, anti-fungal, anti-bacterial, anti-spasmodic, neuroprotectant
❈ Lavender, Amnesia Haze, Headband, Great White Shark, Black Mamba, Skywalker, Death Star OG

Geranyl acetate

+ Citronella, Lemongrass, Sassafras, Rose
))) Floral, Fruity
🌡 473°F, 245°C
⚕ anti-microbial
❈ Headband, Gelato, Orange Cookies

α-humulene

+ Hops, Coriander, Basil
))) Hoppy, Earthy
🌡 388°F, 198°C
⚕ anti-bacterial, pain relief
❈ Girl Scout Cookies, White Widow, Sour Diesel, Durban Poison, Grand Daddy Purple, Kush Group

These statements have not been evaluated by the FDA and are not intended to diagnose, treat or cure any disease. Always check with your physician before starting a new dietary supplement program.

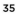 **Terpenes and Testing** Magazine

CBD Living

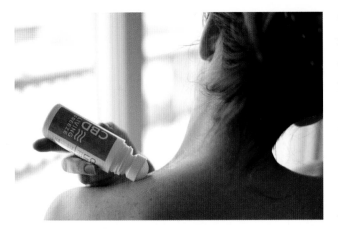

Coming from the medical marijuana industry, Bill D. had a deep understanding of natural, plant-based medicines, so it was a smooth transition when he decided to focus on the CBD business. When he was starting the company, Bill was inspired by all of the personal calls and emails he received on a weekly basis from people sharing their stories on how CBD had changed their lives.

Although CBD is most often incorporated in oils and edibles, the idea of adding it to water was a novel approach that required some sophisticated technology to perfect. It took several years and many scientists and biochemists to create the product that Bill had envisioned. The result of the company's extensive research and development effort was CBD Living Water. The water is a scientific formulation that relies on nano technology to breakdown the CBD particles into nano molecules.

By utilizing this unique manufacturing process, it reduces the CBD oil into nano-sized small droplets, which allows the CBD to more easily pass through the intestinal barrier resulting in enhanced delivery of CBD into the body. Moreover, it allows for a more consistent dose of CBD to be delivered into the body to optimize the health benefits of CBD and homeostasis (balance) in the body.

"It's good for everybody, but our target market initially was children and elders who were looking for a healthier alternative medicine without the psychoactive effect," says Bill.

CBD Living's proprietary technology gives its products increased bioavailability and enhanced absorption, with no chemicals or emulsifiers added. CBD Living Water is always perfectly clear, tasteless, odorless, crisp and clean. The flagship product was a such an early and resounding success that CBD Living soon started formulating other products that incorporated

CBD, including chocolates, gummies, gel caps and topicals.

Launched in 2015, CBD Living's products are now sold in more than 2,000 retail locations including health food stores, medical offices, gyms, dispensaries, and smoke shops. The company has several distribution and production facilities located across the country, and its products can be shipped across the U.S., and are sold internationally.

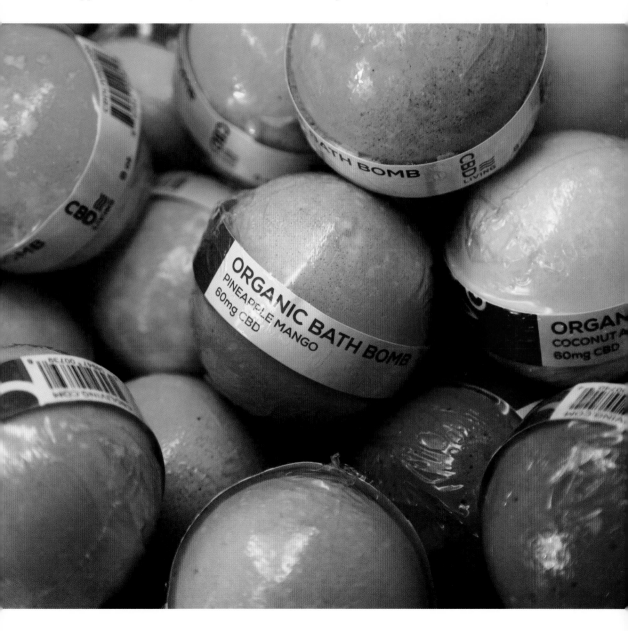

Isodiol International

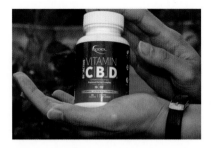

Isodiol International is a Vancouver-based company that produces 99 percent (plus) pure, bioactive pharmaceutical grade cannabinoids, and is an industry leader in the manufacturing and development of phytoceutical consumer products for the pharmaceutical, nutraceutical and cosmetic markets.

The company's mission is to introduce the global population to the importance of endocannabinoid system (ECS) health by providing the highest quality phytocannabinoid-rich products possible. Isodiol International also wants to provide people in need with a product that is natural, non-synthetic and non-toxic in lieu of synthetic pharmaceutical drugs that may have negative side effects. The company's CBD products are made from industrially-cultivated hemp from its cultivation partners and its cannabinoid extracts include crystalline, oils and concentrates.

Many of Isodiol's signature products have been developed by, or in consultation with, medical doctors and scientists who have used these formulas in their practices. Isodiol International's product formulations focus on bioactivity and bioavailability, which means they are meant to work well and work fast. Its products are made with only the highest quality ingredients and work by either systemic or non-systemic interaction with the body's endocannabinoid system to promote homeostasis and balance.

In 2011, the company developed Cebediol™, which was a micro-encapsulation of ISO99™ anhydrous hemp oil specifically designed for greater absorption and effect in topical formulations. Two years of clinical studies were performed on an anti-aging serum made with Cebediol™.

As demand for hemp-derived phytocannabinoid-rich products continues to grow globally, so too does the demand for new delivery systems, including water soluble products such as bottled water, nutrient-enriched beverages, energy shorts, gummies and more. Recognizing this opportunity, in 2014 Isodiol created NanoUltra™, a nanoemulsified anhydrous hemp oil suspended in water and shortly thereafter created HenePlex™, a full spectrum nanoemulsified phytocannabinoid complex suspended in water.

Isodiol has never rested on its laurels, and has been on a steady growth path with its products over the years, adding several divisions and new consumer brands to its portfolio.: IsoBev, founded in 2017, features the Pot-o-Coffee brand; The CBDXtreme division develops consumer products specifically branded for c-stores, smoke & vape shops and dispensaries; and the IsoSport division creates consumer products specifically formulated for the "prosumer athlete."

In 2017, Isodiol International was formed and went public on the CSE (ISOL), OTCQB (ISOLF) and FWB (LW6A). After its public offering, Isodiol International turned its focus towards vertical integration, international expansion and strategic acquisitions of several additional established brands in key market verticals.

The company is now vertically integrated and owns state-of-the-art processing facilities in multiple countries. Additionally, Isodiol International controls an invaluable portfolio of intellectual property including three pivotal processing patents and numerous delivery system patents.

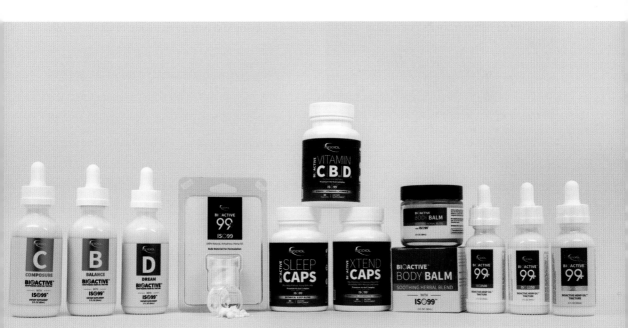

Advanced Nutrients

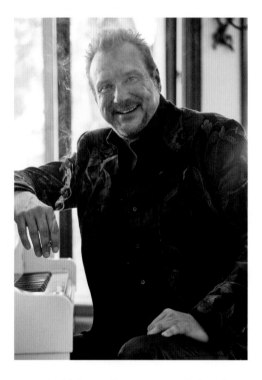

The indelible imprint Advanced Nutrients has left on the cannabis industry is the legacy of company founder BigMike Straumietis, who went from a major player in the North American cannabis cultivation community, to the dynamic force behind the top cannabis growing system and supplement company in the world. Advanced Nutrients is the No. 1 company of its kind, with operations throughout North America, Eastern Europe, Germany and Spain that drive more than $100 million in yearly sales from 100 countries.

The dramatic story of BigMike's career in the underground market is the stuff of movies. Think high-tech counter-surveillance, airplane crashes, assumed identities, cat-and-mouse games with law enforcement, and showdowns with outlaw biker gangs — all against the backdrop of hundreds of millions of dollars and a metric ton of marijuana. Advanced Nutrients has earned global market dominance through tireless dedication to developing scientifically sound, cannabis-specific solutions for cultivators.

Using its government-licensed medical cannabis research facility in Eastern Europe, Advanced Nutrients has invested nearly two decades of intensive research into developing pharmaceutical-grade cannabis nutrients, supplements and cannabinoid research that unlocks the full genetic potential of cannabis for medical or adult use. With a team of 25 Ph.D.'s working around the clock, the team is responsible for more than 50 cannabis research firsts and a line of products that repeatedly win grow competitions the world over.

At a time when hydroponics companies were distancing themselves from cannabis and pretending their products were for growing "tomatoes" or "roses," Advanced Nutrients was the first and only company to create a complete cannabis growing system that takes care of all phases of plant development, from seed to senescence.

The way BigMike saw it, those other companies were profiting from cannabis growers — and they knew it — but they weren't offering specialized support for those high-value grows. It was this desire to create an optimum nutrient solution for the distinct needs of the cannabis grower that ultimately led to the top-selling, award-winning line of products Advanced Nutrients offers today.

Anyone who's interacted with cannabis or the cannabis industry has benefited from one of the many contributions made by BigMike and Advanced Nutrients. And anyone who's ever grown using the clinically proven products from Advanced Nutrients knows what makes the company special — it's in the results.

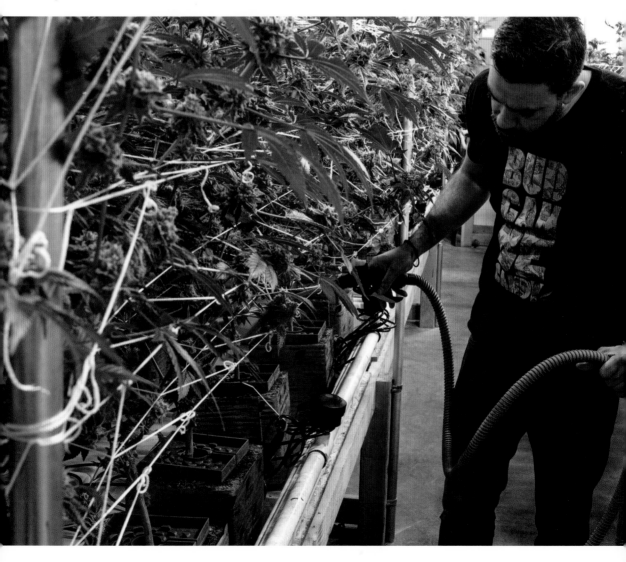

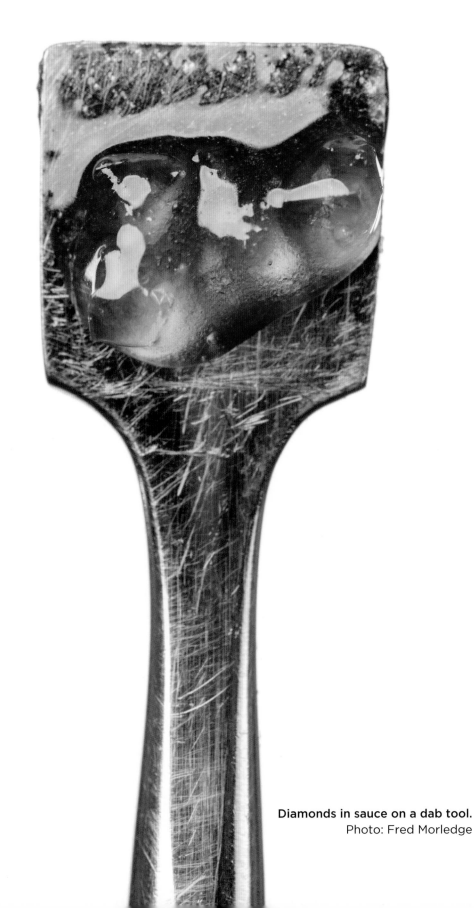

Diamonds in sauce on a dab tool.
Photo: Fred Morledge

CHAPTER 2

Dabbing & Vaping

The Art (and Science) of Consuming Cannabis

There had to be a first lucky human who discovered the intoxicating powers of cannabis. Perhaps this early hominid collecting tinder and kindling inadvertently snatched up a few sticks of sativa and tossed them on the fire, realizing the powerful effects the smoke had only after awaking to the grisly evidence he'd eaten an entire antelope the night before.

Once humans discovered the power of cannabis we immediately poured our collective energy into harnessing it. Archaeologists in Russia uncovered 2,400-year-old, solid-gold bongs used by Scythian chieftains, who thankfully didn't clean their pipes too often, leaving behind resin that confirmed they were indeed used for cannabis. This is the oldest confirmed cannabis pipe discovered, but we know from historical records that chillums and bongs have their roots in pre-antiquity — we've been finding new ways to consume cannabis for as long as we've been using it.

Anyone reading this book is likely familiar with the foundational methods of inhaling cannabis. Most of them are variations on smoking: pipes and joints, many with novelty features. Despite the countless variations, smoking is always fundamentally the same; plant material is set on fire, the process of combustion decarboxylates the cannabinoids, and the resulting smoke is inhaled into the lungs where it enters the bloodstream directly, circumventing the GI tract and heading directly to the brain. Even when it comes to smoking hash, there weren't many major changes in the method for generations; set it on fire and inhale it, not advanced science — until the advent of vaporizers.

A common source of confusion is that the terms *vaping* and *dabbing* get used somewhat interchangeably, for example, when somebody refers to a portable vaporizer used for concentrates as a "dab pen." Some of that confusion is the result of marketing, some of it is because we're dealing with emerging terms and practices that are still being absorbed by the broader cannabis culture. By the end of this chapter you should be fully versed in the various noncombustion options for inhaling cannabis. To start, here's a basic set of parameters:

- The terms *dabbing* and *vaporizing* encompass all the noncombustion methods for inhaling cannabis.
- Vaporizing refers to any noncombustion method for inhaling cannabis; dabbing is a form of vaporizing. However, it can only be applied to concentrates — you cannot dab buds or unpressed kief. So any noncombustion method of inhaling buds or unpressed kief can be accurately termed vaporizing.
- You can dab concentrates, but there are other methods of vaporization that also work. Any noncombustion method of inhaling concentrates can technically be considered vaporizing, but depending on the gear used may more accurately be called dabbing.
- There is some overlap between cannabis and nicotine vaping gear and equipment, but it's always best to use devices specialized for (or at least widely and safely used) for cannabis vaporization.

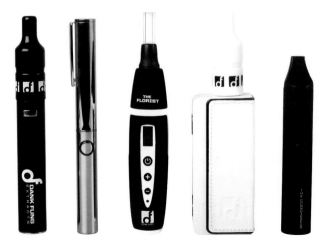

Dank Fung designed their products for the connoisseur. Their wax pen is unique, with no coils and a deep, all-ceramic bowl. The Florist, for bud, also has a ceramic kiln for gentle heating. The rose gold Executive vaporizer is plated with 24 karat gold and has a glass atomizer.

VAPORIZING

Most early adopters of cannabis vaporizing were focused on reducing the harms associated with smoking and the by-products of combustion: Cannabis is an exceptionally safe substance, but burning and inhaling smoke is not a lung-friendly practice. The concept of vaporizing is to activate and release the cannabinoids and terpenes but leave the inert plant matter unburned.

In a way, the practice of vaporizing buds is rooted in the same basic idea behind extraction; accessing the cannabinoids and terpenes without consuming the inactive and potentially harmful plant material. The method of consumption targets desirable elements for vaporization at temperatures too low to combust the plant matter.

The first wave of products created to achieve this or attempt it were inconvenient to use. Few products from this era remain, notwithstanding a few originals on the shelves of smoke shops with nostalgic or optimistic owners. The first was the Tilt Pipe: It resembled a desktop gumball machine, but instead of candy, the glass dome housed a small metal dish that heated up. Put the bud in the dish, turn it on, and inhale warm, bud-flavored air through a length of rubber aquarium tubing. It had fans but never really took off. Why? Inefficient conduction and the War on Drugs, which forced may early cannabis entrepreneurs from the business.

CONDUCTION VS. CONVECTION

All vaporization is characterized by the absence of combustion, the chemical process behind "burning." This largely self-sustaining process is a simple molecular exchange in which carbon is oxidized, yielding carbon dioxide.

Because inhalation of the resulting smoke, while pleasurable, isn't ideal from a respiratory health standpoint, some cannabis consumers prefer methods that provide the instant impact and easy titration of inhalation while reducing contact with harmful smoke. Because heat is required to achieve decarboxylation, some kind of heat transfer is required. There are three kinds: conduction, convection, and radiation. No practical method of vaporization utilizes radiation, so we'll focus on the first two.

CONDUCTION

Conduction is used in vape domes; the material is placed on the heating element, which transfers heat through direct contact — the same way an electric stove heats a skillet. This type of heating works well for concentrates because they melt and continuously recycle the surface area in contact with the heating element. For example, the coil in a reloadable "dab pen," which in its earliest incarnation was physically very similar to the BC Vape, down to the (albeit much smaller) glass dome. But at this early point in the history of vaporizing cannabis, people were more or less exclusively vaping buds. And because conduction relies on direct contact with the material being vaporized, it isn't particularly efficient for dry herbs, which offer limited and static surface area.

However, some popular contemporary dry herb vaporizers, for instance the the Firefly series of portable dry herb and concentrate vapes, use conduction to great effect.

CONVECTION

Vaporizers that use convective heating, which transfers heat from the heating element to the target through the movement of hot air, proved immensely popular as soon as they were introduced and created the widespread embrace of vaporization as a new consumption method.

Rather than heat the cannabis directly using a heating element, convection vaporizers heat the air surrounding the cannabis. When the air reaches the right temperature, it activates and releases the cannabinoids and terpenes without burning the plant material, because the temperature never gets hot enough to create a burn. Convection avoids the charring associated with combustion, making it one of the safest ingestion methods for cannabis inhalation.

The earliest models, such as the Hot Box, were the first of many similar devices; a glass chamber attached to a rubber tube was filled with ground buds, placed in contact with a glass heating element that allowed for air to pass through it when the user inhaled, heating the air and the bud, vaporizing the terps and cannabinoids. Eventually models were released that used forced air and "vape bags." This accelerated the vaporization craze into overdrive.

One enduring favorite from this phase in the evolution of the vaporizer is the Volcano from Storz and Bickel. This was many people's first introduction to vaporization. Ground buds or hash is placed on a specialized screen inside a chamber that was fitted to a plastic bag and placed on a heating element at the top of the conical volcano shape that gives the device its name. The bag fills with vapor thanks to the combined efforts of the heating element and an internal fan, which pushes the vapor into the bag. The bag is fitted with a one-way valve so it can be passed around like a joint and several people can vaporize together. This was the gold standard in vaporizers for a long time and it still has many adherents.

But there is also the new generation of convective vaping devices, which seek to replicate the best parts of the smoking experi-

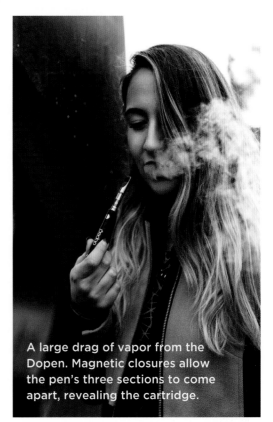

A large drag of vapor from the Dopen. Magnetic closures allow the pen's three sections to come apart, revealing the cartridge.

ence — like taking a full hit from a water pipe — using the benefits of vaporization. One notable standout is the Vapexhale Evo, a system that provides a compact heating base that interlocks with multiple customizable attachments, including basic tube water pipes and more elaborate percolators.

THE BROAD POPULARITY OF VAPING

Why has vaping become so popular? There are many excellent reasons people might choose vaping over smoking.

- **Acceptance** — Many places that specifically forbid smoking allow vapers to fire up their pipes and pens.
- **Portability** — Vape pens and pipes are usually much less bulky than a pack of cigarettes. One slips neatly into a pocket or purse.
- **Convenience** — Vape pens hold a supply of oil or wax that can last for a while.
- **Health considerations** — It's still up for debate as to whether vaping is actually safer than smoking cannabis, but some evidence suggests that this might be the case. In any event, if people believe it's healthier, it could be a factor in vaping's popularity.
- **Popularity** — This might seem a little counterintuitive, but popularity is contagious. People are much more likely to start vaping if it's trendy.

VAPING OIL, WAX, AND DRY HERB – KNOW THE DIFFERENCE

Most vape pipes consist of a rechargeable lithium-ion battery, a heating coil, a chamber, and the apparatus casing that holds it all together. There are three main types of vape pipes and pens:

- Oil
- Dab wax
- Dry herb

All of these vaporizers work by heating the substance that you put into the chamber, whether that's an oil cartridge, wax, or dried cannabis. The heat causes the substance to release a mist that you inhale through the mouthpiece. There are some vape pipes and pens with interchangeable attachments for each substance. You should make sure that you follow the manufacturer's guidelines with regard to the type of vape substance you put in your pipe or pen.

As with any other purchase, you should do your own research to determine what the best vape pens and vape pipes are. Make sure you pick one that's made for the type of substance that you want to vape.

DABBING

Consuming cannabis through inhalation is an ancient practice, so there aren't too many truly new ideas when it comes to getting the active ingredients into your lungs. Still, it's hard to point to a more revolutionary shift in contemporary cannabis consumption than the one that's grown out of the emergence of dabbing. Concentrates used to serve a supporting role to the undeniable "star" of the cannabis market, raw buds. Now, with the widespread embrace of dabbing, concentrates have taken center stage in the commercial and cultural conversation around cannabis. The practice has also been instrumental in shifting the focus of connoisseurs from cannabinoid potency to terpene profiles.

WHAT'S A DAB?

Dabbing is a way to consume large amounts of terpenes, THC, and other cannabinoids, while radically reducing unhealthy pyrolitic compounds.

It's hard to pin down the precise origins of the word *dab*. The prevailing assumption is that it was inspired (at least indirectly) by the marketing slogan for the early 20th Century hair dressing Brylcreem; "A little dab'll do ya," the implication in both instances being that very little product is needed to achieve the desired effect.

WHEN LESS IS MORE

With high-potency cannabis concentrates, a person can experience the effects of smoking an entire joint or more in a single breath, using only enough product to cover a pinhead. Think of it as the difference between drinking beer and liquor: If you drink a standard can or bottle of beer with an ABV of 5%, you're drinking 12 ounces of liquid but less than an ounce of actual alcohol; if you drink a typical "shot" of 80-proof spirits, you're only consuming 0.6 ounces of alcohol, but you're also only drinking 1.5 ounces of liquid.

The complex suite of cannabinoids, terpenes, and other active compounds found in the cannabis plant affect the human body through a more sophisticated biological mechanism than ethanol, so side-by-side comparison between raw buds and concentrates can't be done quite as precisely as beer and liquor. But conceptually speaking, it's a solid foundation for understanding their relative potencies: You might drink a 12-ounce beer at a picnic, but you (probably) wouldn't chug half a fifth of vodka — and if you did, you'd almost certainly regret it, even though you'd be consuming roughly the same volume of liquid. In the same way, you might be able to take a massive bong rip of raw buds, but trying to use the same approach for your first dab could result in an unpleasant experience. If you keep this in mind when dosing your dabs, you'll avoid the potential discomfort and anxiety of overloading your senses.

DABBING: THE PROCESS

Dabbing is a relatively simple process, but unlike vaporization, highly concentrated material is required: There's no way to dab buds. In fact, the primary physical trait that makes a concentrate "dabbable" is the absence of plant material and the high concentration of cannabinoids and terpenes.

So truly full-melt hash or high-grade hashish can be lightly pressed and dabbed — really oily hash presses out into a dabbable patty with some gentle kneading pressure using your palm and the thumb of your opposite hand. Hash can also be pressed into rosin, which is also dabbable. All solvent-extracted concentrates are dabbable.

There are various ways to take a dab, but they all rely on the same basic principle: a heating element is brought to the ideal temperature for activating cannabinoids and evaporating terpenes. Cannabis concentrate is placed on the heating element, and the heat creates vapor which is inhaled.

Because dabbing utilizes highly potent concentrates, the effects can be felt immediately. For some people, this makes it a more effective treatment for pain, anxiety and other conditions that call for quick relief.

Dabbing is a conductive method of vaporing concentrates because the heating element makes direct contact with the material being inhaled. If the temperature of the heating element is too high, then the concentrates are combusting. This defeats the purpose of dabbing and exposes you to potentially harmful chemicals. However, when done correctly, dabbing will boil the concentrate, allowing for inhalation of the resulting vapor.

To understand the process of dabbing, it helps to first understand its crude predecessor; hot knifing hash.

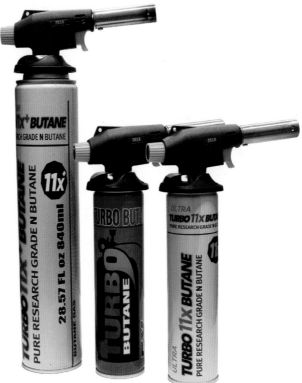

Zilla's Twist-on-Torch will fit most butane canister brands and sizes. It has adjustable air and gas intake and flame control.

HOT KNIFING: THE DIRTY OLD GRANDPA OF DABBING

Hot Knifing was the first method of dabbing. It isn't high tech; it uses tools found in the kitchen. Here's the basic technique for hot knifing. The method uses at least one very hot knife.

MATERIALS NEEDED

- Two dinner knives that won't be missed
- A hollow bamboo, cardboard or metal tube. Don't use plastic because of possible off-gassing.
- A heat source such as torch or stovetop
- Concentrate: Hash is easiest because it's less likely to melt and drip.
- Scissors

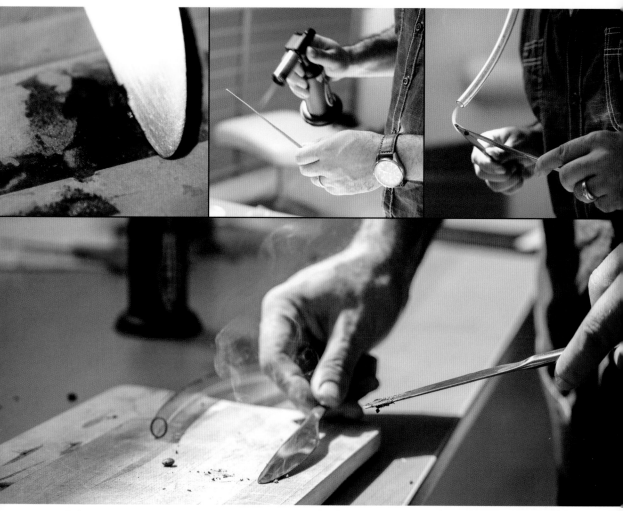

Top: Scraping recently heated and pressed hash onto a cold knife. Heating a second knife with a butane torch. By pressing the hot knife on to the decarboxylated hash, vapor is created.
Bottom: Hash vapor rising from a warm knife as Greg Zeman prepairs for another dab.
Photos: Lizzy Fritz

STEPS

1. Heat one of the knives. This can be done by placing the blade in the flame of a torch or gas stove, or by wedging it into an electric stove's heating coil.

2. Prepare a vapor collection funnel by using a long cardboard tube from a spent roll of paper towels or a metal or wooden straw.

3. Gently heat the other knife using the stove or a lighter — just enough to make the hash stick to it without burning off.

3A. With concentrates use a teaspoon to hold the oil, wax, or shatter and dip the hot knife into it.

4. If alone, take one knife in each hand and flatten the tube to make a mouthpiece and hold it in your mouth. If flat ironing with more than one person, a friend can assist the smoker, allowing the smoker to simply hold the tube.

5. Position the collection funnel over the two knives and press them together, squishing the hash between the blades. Take care not to let them touch the funnel.

6. Time your breath to inhale as much of the cloud of smoke created as possible.

7. Repeat process as required.

This works, but it isn't a health-conscious practice; the potential for inhaling chemicals from the knives, the possibility of burns, and the inefficient use of hash make it a less than ideal method. Historically, it laid the conceptual groundwork for dabbing.

A WORD ON HOT DABS

Hot dabs are how most dabbers were introduced to dabbing, but thankfully this is no longer a necessary rite of passage now that low-temp dabbing has become the majority practice. It isn't just that hot dabs hurt when you take them, they can hurt you in the long run.

A recent study conducted by Portland State University's chemistry department — one of the first to explore the effects of terpenoid degradation in the context of cannabis concentrate consumption — found that dabs over 750°F (400°C) degrees can contribute to the formation of carcinogen-filled smoke, and that even hotter dabs present an even greater risk.

The study, led by PSU chemistry professor Robert Strongin, showed that oils present in the extract release potentially cancer-causing chemicals when heated to temperatures above 750°F. When heated above 932°F, oils released benzene, a known carcinogen.

LOW-TEMP DABS — THE FIRST CLASS TICKET TO TERP TOWN

The key to effective dabbing is finding the ideal balance between preserving the terpenes while activating the cannabinoids. The problem is that the volatization point of most terpenes is far below the boiling point of most cannabinoids. Compromises must be made. Lower temps mean higher terps and fewer activated cannabinoids, higher temps mean lower terps and higher cannabinoid activation. While the boiling point of THC is generally said to be 315°F, that number is actually the boiling point in a low-pressure environment. The boiling point of THC at normal atmospheric pressure probably falls somewhere between 350°F and 400°F, too hot at the top end to preserve terps. Thankfully, low-temp dabs utilize low pressure, achieved through restricted airflow via a carb cap.

Carb caps can be as simple as a flat, glass surface with a hole in it and as complex as a "directional" cap with an angled vent built into it, but the point is the same; it restricts and directs airflow, lowering the pressure and by extension the boiling points of both the terpenes and cannabinoids present. This allows for a flavorful, low-temp dab that still contains high levels of active cannabinoids.

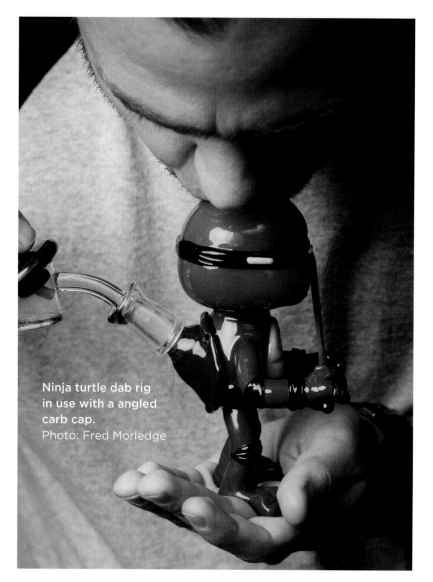

Ninja turtle dab rig
in use with a angled
carb cap.
Photo: Fred Morledge

HOW TO TAKE A LOW-TEMP DAB

While a laser thermometer can be used to precisely target certain temperatures, it isn't really necessary to be that precise when it comes to enjoying a low-temp dab. If you do decide to use a laser thermometer, you'll want to dial in a temperature that's somewhere between 315°F and 450°F — the optimum range for activation of cannabinoids and preservation of terpenes. The specific temperature target will ultimately depend on your preference and the idiosyncrasies of the product being consumed, but anything in this range should provide a potent, flavorful vapor. There are some dabbers who still use ceramic or titanium heating elements, but for optimum flavor the best choice is quartz glass, which will not alter the taste of your dab.

Regardless of what style of "nail" or "banger" you use, the basics are the same — these directions assume you're using a torch rather than an e-nail.

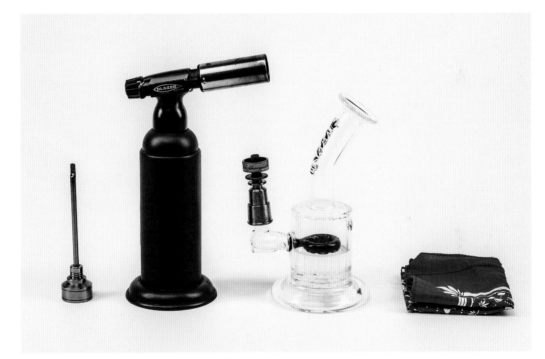

Tools for dabbing: dab tool or stick with attached carb cap, torch, dab right with titanium nail, and dab rag, for cleaning your sticky tools when your finished.
Photo: Fred Morledge

- Heat the nail until the bottom begins to glow faintly orange. It doesn't have to be even; the point is to establish a visual "cue" so that you're heating it to roughly the same temperature each time.

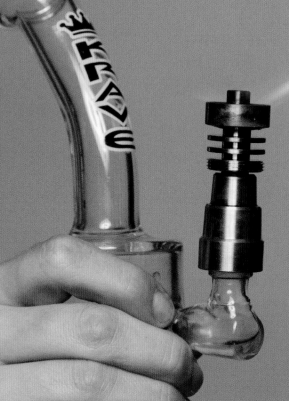

The proper distance for heating a nail:
The core flame just touches the nail.

A red-hot nail alerts the
dabber that the temperature
is hot enough. It will need to
cool before placing the dab.

- Wait — the length of waiting time can range from 15 to more than 60 seconds depending on the nail/banger used and the initial heat level. If you have a heat gun, you can expedite the "dialing in" process, but may need to find the sweet spot through trial and error. The key is to have it hot enough to create dense vapor when capped, but not so hot as to leave scorch marks on the glass afterward. People often employ timers once they've dialed in the ideal cooling-off period.

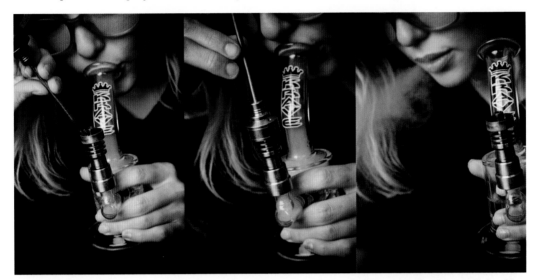

After placing the dab on your dab tool, place the tool and dab onto the hot nail, begin to inhale. Cover the cap onto the nail after the dab has melted onto it to retain all the vapor. Exhale immediately, it's not good for your lung health to hold hot dab vapor in.
Photos: Fred Morledge

- Place your dab in the banger using a dab tool and cap using the carb cap — you know what to do next — now exhale.
- Wipe out any residual extract using a cotton swab. Again, if you've done it right, the banger should wipe clean.
- Repeat as needed/desired.

You'll know you did it right when taking a dab tastes the way the source material smells.

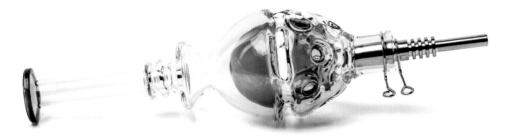

The Faberge Egg Dab Straw by Pulsar is Swiss cut glass that includes a titanium nail and is 11 inches long. The Faberge egg-shaped body swirls and cools the vapor.
Photo: Fred Morlege

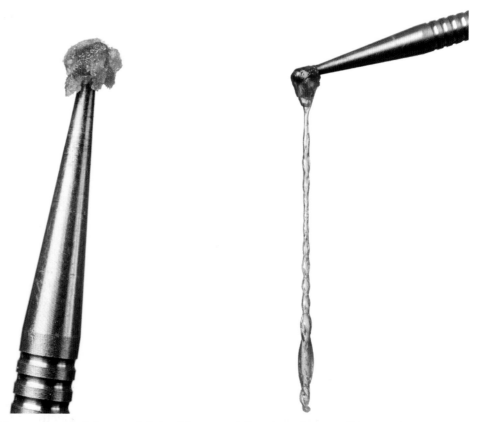

A small to moderate dab on a dab tool is around the size of a pencil led to the eraser. Larger dabs are often excessive and wasteful, be prepared to take multiple breaths.
Photos: Fred Morlege

DANGERS OF DABBING

Dabbing has an inherently dangerous look to it, and that may be part of the attraction for some dabbers. Butane torches put people off, as do the red-hot nails and the sight of strange-looking substances boiling off into glassware. Many people consider dab culture a liability to the overall legalization of marijuana, noting how the media have dubbed it "the crack" of pot. The analogy is incorrect. Dabs are more like the espresso or hard liquor of pot.

Unlike liquor, there is no lethal dose for marijuana. However, you can pass out from smoking bud or dabbing. THC lowers blood pressure, so dab sitting down whenever possible. Overdosing on THC, while not dangerous, can be uncomfortable, causing anxiety and even nausea.

DABBING DOS AND DON'TS

- Don't dab unless you're an experienced cannabis user.
- Don't make dabbing a contest.
- Do small dabs and enjoy yourself. Huge dabs increase your tolerance, can result

in acute intoxication, and can be part of a constellation of behaviors that could ultimately lead to harm.

- Keep temperatures as low as possible to vaporize extracts.
- Sudden exposure to very hot, dry air can cause your throat to close up, as though you were choking. Prevent any physiological damage to your lungs and throat by using a pipe cooled with water or ice.
- Use care and common sense when operating a torch, as well as handling potentially hot nails, wands, and other heating elements used in dabbing.

ELECTRIC DABS: THE EVOLUTION OF DAB CULTURE AND TECH

Most people seem to agree dabbing hit the cannabis mainstream around 2009. Everything changed; what started as an underground movement became a dominant thread. Now dab culture is no longer an outlier of cannabis culture: it's one of the driving forces of its evolution. The practice of dabbing fuels the demand for dabbable products, which drives the development of new technologies and practices for creating better and stronger concentrates.

Dabbing, like most new things, is somewhat controversial: Some consider the use of torches a public relations liability for the cannabis decriminalization movement at a pivotal cultural moment. And while many people appreciate the intense flavors and effects of a dab, others are put off by the potency and immediacy compared to smoking buds.

Concentrates surged in popularity in the medical marijuana epicenters and are spreading. Dispensaries that once carried a shelf of water hash now feature concentrates. At cannabis festivals, the once-ubiquitous vapor bags for large groups have disappeared, replaced by electric dab rigs and bud baristas doling out dab after dab to an endless line of enthusiasts. Pre-rolls and bong hits were once the mainstay of cannabis festival giveaways; free dabs are the complimentary coin of the realm now.

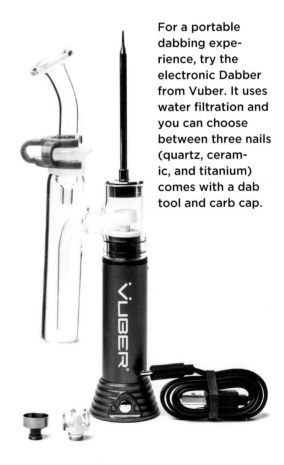

For a portable dabbing experience, try the electronic Dabber from Vuber. It uses water filtration and you can choose between three nails (quartz, ceramic, and titanium) comes with a dab tool and carb cap.

E-NAILS

Many people are turned off by the butane torch, which looks industrial and primitive at the same time. E-nails heat a nail using electricity rather than a flame. Plug-in or battery-powered electric heating elements affix to a nail and heat it up in seconds. The best thing about an e-nail is the consistent temperature, which allows for bigger dabs and more efficient use of the material. Unlike a torch dab, which results in the heating element cooling fairly rapidly, the steady heat of an e-nail allows for full consumption of the entire dab, leaving no residue.

The typical e-nail is composed of a controller, which houses the digital temperature readout and the electrical components. A detachable cord attaches to the unit on one end, terminating in a metal heating coil on the other. In terms of temperature, you'll be able to dial it in precisely on the digital readout every e-nail has, but remember that the temperature setting is the temperature of the coil, so assume the temperature of the banger or nail is slightly lower.

E-nails are the future of dabbing.

Ready to dab out of the box, The Colorado Native Hive set has a rig with over 100 holes of percolation and has zero drag with spiraling water tornados during every dab. The set includes the temperature control box that has dual usb ports, 22mm Kevlar wrapped heating coil (5 ft long) that fits all of the Bee Nails, like the one included in this kit with the silicone dab mat, carb cap, and dab container. Photo: Fred Morledge

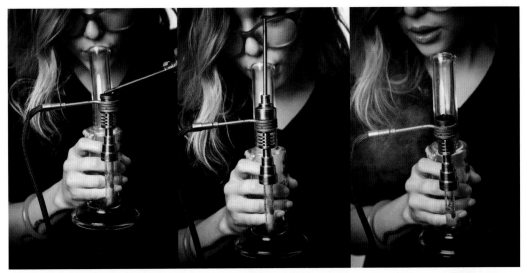

Dabbing with an e-nail is the same as dabbing with a torch, but is seen as safer since there is no flame and the temperature can me more accurately set to low temp dabs. Most nails are quite fast to heat up and can be left on safely. Place the dab on your tool and add it to the nail, cover with a carb cap, while inhaling remove the cap and clear the rig of its vapor. Photos: Fred Morledge

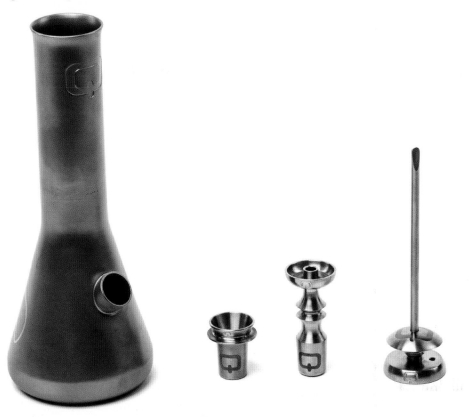

When you don't want your rig to break: Quiver Fabrications has made the Grade 1 Titanium rig set. It includes the Kenai concentrate nail that is designed for low-temp use and quick heat up / cool down times. Photo: Fred Morledge

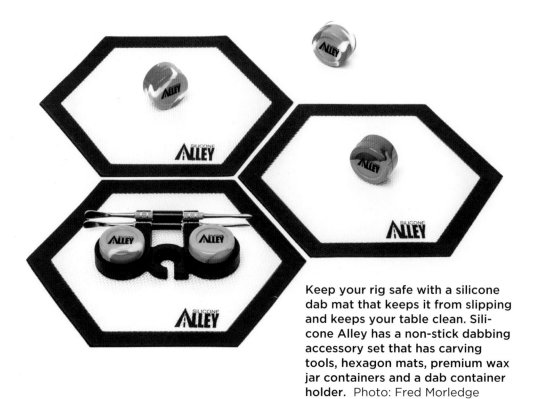

Keep your rig safe with a silicone dab mat that keeps it from slipping and keeps your table clean. Silicone Alley has a non-stick dabbing accessory set that has carving tools, hexagon mats, premium wax jar containers and a dab container holder. Photo: Fred Morledge

DABBING — THE GEAR

If you're new to dabbing, the abundance of different techniques and technologies available can be overwhelming — everything from consumption devices to containers comes in a dozen different styles and can be constructed from several different materials. What do you really need when it comes to dabbing gear and what are the best options? Regardless of what gear you use, the basic criteria for your choice are the same; having accounted for your budget, what available option will provide the most flavorful and effective dabbing experience?

While everything in cannabis consumption ultimately boils down to personal preference, there are some methods that have fallen out of popular use because more efficient options are now available. There's no accounting for all outliers and personal preferences, so we've tried to provide as many options as possible, and where applicable, we've highlighted the most desirable and/or popular ones.

One example of the way dabbing gear has evolved is the evolution of the heating elements used, now often referred to as "nails" or "bangers." Whether you use a torch or an electric coil to heat them, these are arguably the centerpiece of the dabbing experience: You can spend top dollar on a fancy dab rig with a dozen percolators, but if you take your dab too hot or too cold the experience will be far from premium — even less so if the banger is made from subpar materials that leach potentially harmful chemicals into your dab.

When dabbing first emerged, the heating was largely done using metal, specifically titanium — the only metal safe to use for dabbing, thanks to its exceptionally low "outgassing property." This means that, unlike other metals, it will not release toxic chemicals at the relatively high heats used for dabbing, making it the obvious choice for dabbing off metal.

Titanium was and still is prized by some dabbers for its unbreakable durability, but even those who still swear by titanium nails will generally acknowledge that the flavor isn't quite as clean as dabbing off ceramic or quartz; there's a faint metallic tinge to everything you dab off titanium, which isn't particularly desirable now that dabbing is focused on experiencing terpene profiles. But when dabbing first started the emphasis was almost entirely on cannabinoid potency. Additionally, everyone was taking hot dabs before the science on low-temp dabbing was fully understood, and titanium retains heat for a relatively long time. Now that low-temp dabs are generally understood to be healthier and more desirable, the even-heating but quick-cooling properties of quartz glass bangers — in addition to the perfectly neutral flavor of a clean one — make it the preferred choice for dab connoisseurs.

But if you do decide to use titanium, it's important to remember that all titanium components are coated with polish during manufacturing and may also have some residual compounds from the factory, so you have to "season" the nail (heat it orange hot and cool it in water several times) to reduce the metallic taste and the potential for ingesting harmful chemicals.

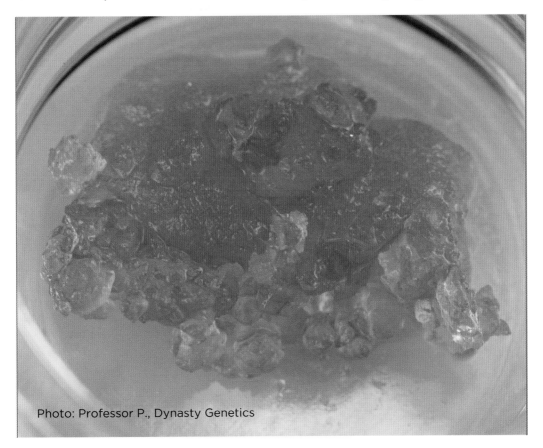

Photo: Professor P., Dynasty Genetics

Ceramic heating elements were also popular for a while, but like titanium they impart a distinct if not unpleasant taste, sometimes compared to the smell of a brick oven or cooking stone. Ceramic is pretty much just as fragile as quartz too, so there's little benefit to its use, apart from reduced cost. When it comes to e-nails, many people do indeed use metal and ceramic, but the new standard is quartz glass bangers, which provide optimum heat and flavor particularly when using a torch. Unlike ceramic and titanium, quartz glass does not require any seasoning.

BANGERS VS. NAILS

Because one of the earliest centerpieces of dab gear was literal titanium nails, the word *nail* still sometimes gets used in a colloquial sense when discussing whatever heating element is used for dabbing. Generally though, particularly in Northern California and other cultural hubs of the dab scene, what's really being discussed is a banger, which roughly amounts to a tiny glass or quartz bucket attached to a downstem for a water pipe.

The banger is heated, then cooled, and concentrate is placed inside it. If the temperature is just right, the cannabinoids and terpenes will boil off into vapor that can be inhaled through whatever pipe or rig the banger is attached to. A low temperature can be compensated for using a carb cap, which lowers the surface tension of the boiling concentrate and allows for higher vapor production. For this reason, there aren't many dab rigs that still come with dome attachments, although they're still floating around, particularly on the cheaper options.

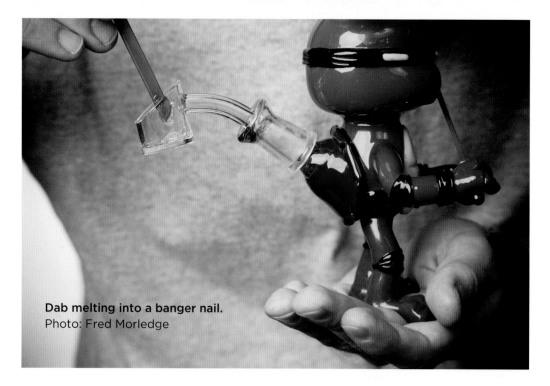

Dab melting into a banger nail.
Photo: Fred Morledge

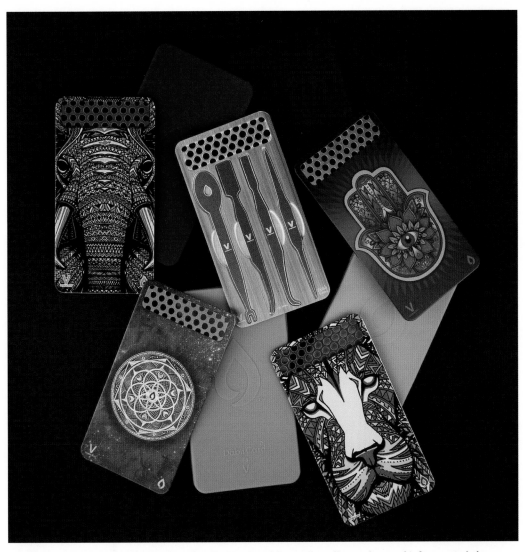

Portable concentrate tool kit: The Debit Card by V Syndicate is made from stainless steel. It can handle a range of concentrates. Housed in a silicone case, your sticky tools won't make a mess. It includes a patented grinder as well.

Nails were the workhorses of the dab world. But now bangers are more popular. They come in a variety of standard widths, like 10 mm, 14 mm, and 18 mm, to fit into different bangers and downstems. Nails are made from a variety of materials that are used because they don't create fumes at working vaporization temperatures. The most common materials used are quartz, titanium, and ceramic.

As covered above, a carb cap makes the rig more efficient. It's placed over the banger immediately after the dab has been dropped on the nail. It prevents the vapor from escaping from the top and slows any burning by making oxygen scarce. It allows for extra-low temperatures and the best flavors. It has replaced the dome, which is scarcely seen anymore.

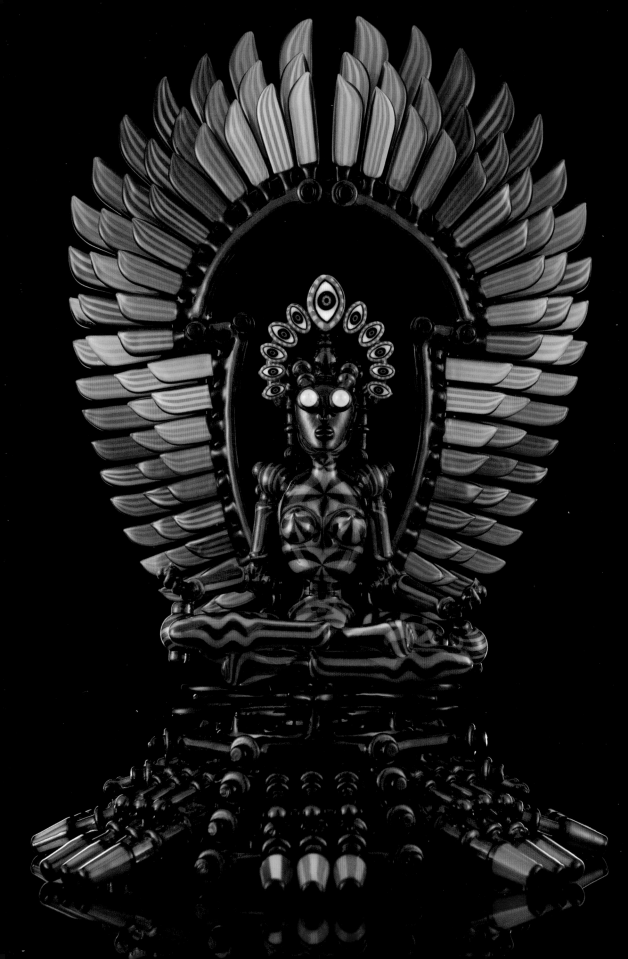

Dab Rigs

While bangers can fit into a wide variety of downstems, they are designed for use with dab rigs, aka bongs and bubblers specially designed for consuming hash.

Dab rigs tend to be smaller than water pipes for flowers. Since hash smoke is much more potent, you don't need to fill a huge chamber with smoke to achieve the desired effect. Solvent hash condenses along the route of delivery, so the longer the route, the more condensation and the more waste: Smaller is better for dab rigs.

Dab rig design is divided into two general classes, scientific and heady, though plenty of artists seek to fuse the two. Scientific designs hew toward a minimalist, lab aesthetic and often feature clear glass and shapes that evoke beakers and test tubes. Form follows function in scientific glass. Scientific dab rigs can get incredibly technical , with multiple levels of diffusers and percolators. Heady dab rig designs embrace the imagination, taking on the shape of mythic creatures and pushing the boundaries of color, pattern, and materials.

Left: Isis Ina Dab Rig – May, 2015 Artist: Banjo Photo: Alex Reyna

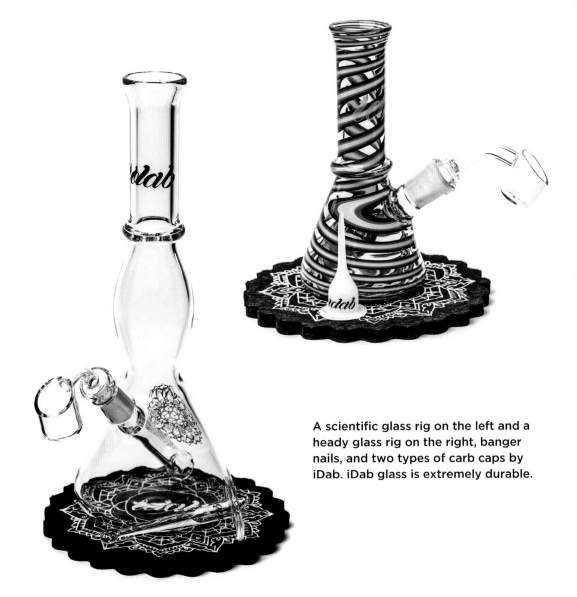

A scientific glass rig on the left and a heady glass rig on the right, banger nails, and two types of carb caps by iDab. iDab glass is extremely durable.

Heady artists are in a permanent arms race for the newest glass colors and coolest-looking designs and materials. Dragons, robots, cartoon characters, and monsters abound. Artists regularly use metallic fuming and bind different elements to the borosilicate glass, creating deep, rich, luminous colors, sparkles, and interference patterns. Some artists use external electroplating for steampunk-like designs. Many artists are incorporating UV and light-reactive or color-changing designs. The artists designing these rigs are creating a new genre of art that will be used in daily life, but also saved as collectibles.

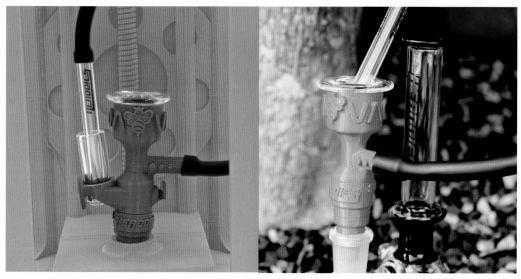

The easy-to-use 3D-Printed DabVac is another innovation from the glass enthusiasts @Headdies! This universal device fits any water-pipe or bubbler turning it into a dabbing machine. The silicone cap and removable dish allows storage without pet hair and dust. Place your wax in the dish, heat the quartz wand for five seconds, and apply the heated tip to the concentrate.

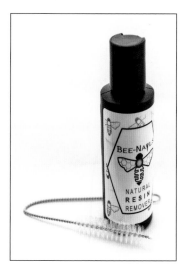

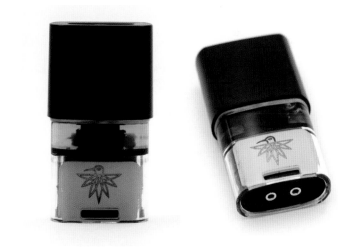

Remove the stickiest resin with Bee-Nails Natural Resin remover. It's made of 100% plant-based oils that are non-toxic, odorless and tasteless. Can be used on glass, metal, ceramic/porcelain, quartz, finished wood, sealed stone, and more.

Live resin cartridges from Harmony Extracts includes cannabis extract and terpenes in various styles of cartridges.

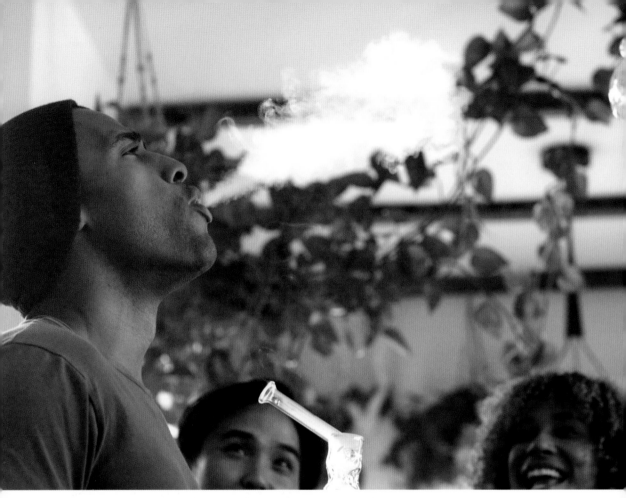

Hitting a Hydratube by Vapexhale. Photo: Vapexhale

VAPORIZERS: WHAT YOU NEED TO KNOW

Dabbing refers to a fairly specific, concentrate-exclusive consumption method, and the gear is largely focused on glassware and accessories for such, with e-nails representing the primary widespread electronic modification to the process. Vaporization, on the other hand, encompasses several approaches to inhaling the active ingredients of buds and extracts, and has evolved along multiple paths, creating a sprawling spectrum of gadgets and gear that many new consumers find overwhelming. How do you pick the right one? What do they actually do? What do I put in them?

We can't make an exhaustive list of the hundreds of products out there, but we've outlined the basic vaporizer types — you already know the different methods for vaporization. We've also compiled some representative product profiles, which cover a wide range of available device types, and explain their capabilities, advantages, and relative disadvantages. It isn't comprehensive, but it should provide a helpful overview of what sorts of options are out there when it comes to vaporizers.

DESKTOP VAPORIZERS

The term *desktop vaporizer* covers a broad suite of stationary devices that plug into an outlet instead of using a battery, which reduces their portability but boosts the power available to their heating elements, allowing for more efficient vaporization and uninterrupted vape sessions of any length. They obviously aren't practical for on-the-go use, but they aren't too large to travel with either. In fact, many cannabis consumers have found that a desktop unit is the perfect travel companion when staying at non smoking hotels; chances are good that you'll still be in violation of their no-smoking policy if you do this, but with even a shred of discretion chances are good that hotel security will never notice.

As with all consumer electronics, there are dozens of stylistic and functional variations available from different manufacturers and models, but when it comes to the practical method of consumption offered by a desktop unit, there are two basic approaches: delayed and immediate inhalation of vapor.

The primary example of delayed inhalation is the old "turkey bag" approach popularized by the Storz and Bickel Volcano. The device forces hot air through a chamber containing cannabis, decarboxylating it and producing an active cannabinoid-rich vapor that is collected inside a plastic bag on the other side of the chamber. Once the bag is filled with vapor, it's removed from the heating base and fitted with an air valve that allows for easy inhalation without any meaningful loss of vapor. The bag can now be passed around like a joint until it's empty, at which point it may be time to repeat the process until the desired effect is achieved.

During active inhalation, the vapor is being consumed as it's made, more akin to a bong rip: The airflow that pulls the smoke or vapor into the consumer's lungs is the same airflow that produces that vapor or smoke. Sometimes that airflow is produced using a simple length of tubing known as a "whip," which attaches directly to the heating element, allowing for immediate inhalation of vapor. Previous generations of vaporizers generally used a single vapor delivery method, but many newer devices allow for both delayed and immediate consumption.

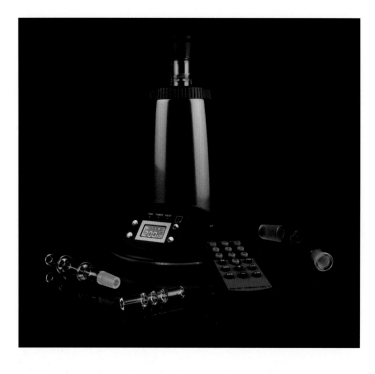

Arizer Extreme Q

Those looking for the classic simplicity of a whip and bag/balloon vaporizer in one unit, with some enhanced features like remote control, will find that the Arizer Extreme Q is a relatively affordable option, with an average retail price of roughly $200.

At 6.7 inches tall and 6.5 inches in diameter, the Extreme Q is a bit on the large side compared with other contemporary desktop vaporizers, but not prohibitively so; it will take up about as much desk space as a small lamp. The clean, industrial design has a fun retro feel, with the innocuous look of a kitchen appliance or an old stereo system component — the inclusion of a remote control with decidedly pre-millennial aesthetics underlines the 1990s hi-fi vibe: It isn't exactly incognito, but it doesn't scream cannabis either.

Using the Extreme Q is fairly simple, and the procedure should be familiar to anyone who's ever used a whip or balloon-style vaporizer: Material is finely ground and placed inside the bowl or chamber, the target temperature is set using the digital temperature readout, and, after 5 minutes or so, the preferred delivery system (whip or balloon) is attached and it's time to vaporize.

You just read one of the main downsides of the Arizer Extreme Q — it takes about 5 minutes to reach target temperature. For some people this isn't an issue, but for those seeking more immediate gratification it may be a little long, particularly when compared with faster heating systems available at a similar price point. There are also many small glass components, making it easy to misplace or break something crucial. And while the remote control seems useful in theory, being able to control the settings from across the room on a device you have to stand directly in front of isn't actually very helpful.

On the plus side, the unit offers both whip and balloon function, adding additional value over single-function devices, and it can also hold up to a half gram of herb in its vape chamber.

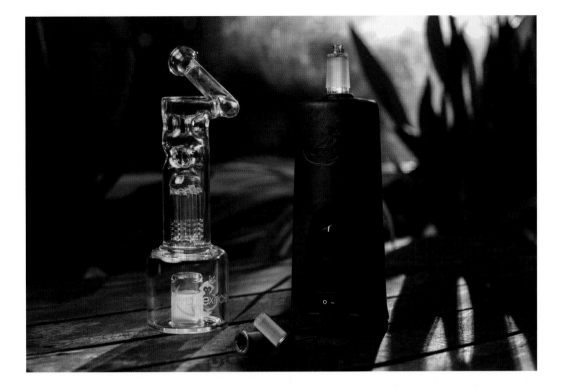

Vapexhale Evo

Whip and balloon systems are an efficient way to inhale cannabis vapor, but some consumers are looking for a vape system that more closely mirrors the sensory experience of hitting a traditional water pipe or dab rig. For them, there's the Vapexhale EVO, which offers both whip-style inhalation and pioneering "Hydratube" attachments, which are basically little bongs that fit on top of the same glass hub the whip would, allowing those used to smoking to take a "rip" like they normally would.

The EVO doesn't just slap fancy glass on top of a convection vaporizer; the heating element of the device has been specifically engineered to replicate the characteristics of a smoked bowl. Most convection vapes have a fatal flaw where vapor volume is concerned; they cool down slightly if you hit harder. As a result, devices require users to tailor their inhalation power to the heating ability of the device, meaning no aggressive "rips." The EVO changes all that with its patented PerpetuHeat technology, which adjusts the heat in response to the rate and force of inhalation. So instead of cooling the heater core, a deep breath will slightly intensify it to compensate, resulting in even vapor production no matter how you hit it.

This advanced heating system, coupled with the glass hydratubes (or your own favorite glass water pipe if you connect it to the EVO using the available adapter) provides a vaporizing experience that matches (and in some ways exceeds) that of a traditional bong bowl, with all the health and flavor benefits of convection vaporizing. Instead of a rubber whip, a short glass tube attachment provides an unfussy, direct vapor path. Additionally, the EVO can handle flower and concentrates beautifully.

The EVO base is small — 6.5 inches tall and 2.5 inches wide — with a subtle, simplistic design built around a knob that turns the device on and sets the temperature. All the way to the left is off; all the way to the right is hot enough to clean the glass chambers used for vaping concentrate and every useful temp in between. It offers one of the best vaping experiences on the market, so the main downside is the relatively high cost, which is still substantially lower than truly expensive devices like the Volcano.

PORTABLE VAPORIZERS

Desktop vaporizers undoubtedly offer many benefits, which is why they continue to enjoy widespread popularity. But much of the buzz around vaporizers is linked to the smaller models, which use battery power to provide discrete, non-combustion cannabis access on the go. Particularly at a time when more and more municipalities and rental complexes are restricting or prohibiting smoking outright, many cannabis enthusiasts are reliant on portable vaporizers to avoid running afoul of those policies, or at least avoid detection.

There's also a rapidly expanding segment of cannabis consumers who live particularly active lifestyles, making a stationary vaporizer impractical: Most people wouldn't consider taking a bong rip at a bus stop or while walking down a city sidewalk, but many might consider surreptitiously hitting a joint or blunt in those same circumstances. In much the same way, portable

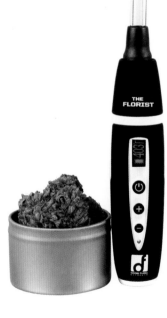

vaporizers provide a low-profile, non-combustion method for enjoying the benefits of inhaled cannabis on the go. As with desktop models, these devices range in price substantially, but because of the smaller quantity of materials used to produce them, a relatively high-end portable vaporizer can be purchased for less than even a mid-range desktop model.

Dank Fung The Florist

Many of the smaller vaporizers rely on conduction — direct contact between the material and the heating element — which compromises the flavor when vaping flowers. The Florist offers the same kind of convection heating used in the desktop models we profiled, but in a handheld device. With precise digital temperature control, the device can be dialed in to maximize the flavor and vapor of your given material, and there's no waiting because you can start inhaling while it heats. The design of the Dank Fung is biased toward terpene retention, so you can count on a flavorful experience, but the USB chargeable battery doesn't have the capacity to last all day, so count on charging it a lot as well.

At 3.2 inches in length, the unit is small enough to fit in the average pocket, and the ceramic heating element provides gentle, even heat for a smooth, dense, flavor-rich vapor. It also offers an affordable option, with an average retail price of $99. On the downside, the small chamber requires frequent reloading and doesn't lend itself well to sharing with others.

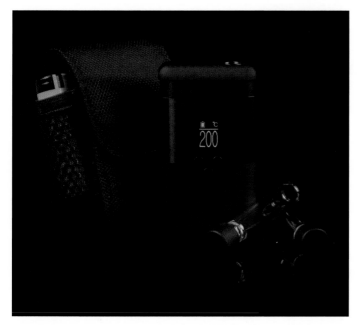

Arizer Go

The Arizer Go, aka ArGo, is a high-end, dry herb vaporizer with several features that allow it to stand out in a very crowded field. Much like Arizer's larger vaporizers, the Air 2 and Solo 2, the ArGo has a vapor-cooling, flavor-preserving, borosilicate glass mouthpiece. Only, this one can be retracted for safety, enhancing the ArGo's already impressive portability. With a price tag nearing $300, the ArGo isn't the cheapest option out there, but its simple design (based on preloadable glass cartridges that pop easily into the device) and precise, reliable heating function make it a standout.

The ArGo is compact and discrete; its boxy, palm-sized design and deliberately nondescript, black finish give it the look of a pager. Even with the retractable glass mouthpiece extended, it looks more like a nicotine vaporizer than something intended for cannabis use, boosting its incognito factor. The precise temperature control and informative OLED display only adds to the device's convenience.

Like most smaller vaporizers, the battery life is short — only about an hour and change — and the vapor production isn't massive. Overall, the ArGo is an attractive and intelligently designed vaporizer, perfect for those focused on high-flavor, low-profile vaping on the go, and there are few products that offer a better experience by that criteria.

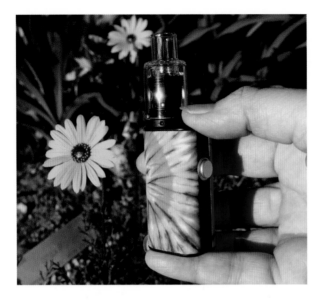

Pulsar APX Wax

Some portable units try to work dry herb and concentrate function into one device, and there are a few standouts in the dual-use category, but when it comes to straightforward, single-function portables with an emphasis on concentrates, the Pulsar APX Wax is a market leader.

With a triple-quartz coil atomizer housed in a pure-quartz heating chamber powered by a long-lasting, quick-charging 1100mAh battery, the small (3.5 inches tall) but powerful APX provides quick, efficient, and flavorful vapor production at the press of a button. And with a price point of $69 retail, the APX offers high value at a low cost. The main downside is that the APX doesn't have adjustable heat — you just push the button and hit it. Given the all-quartz heating element, the flavor is still excellent, but this could be a hard sell for control freaks looking to precisely dial in the ideal temp for each concentrate they vape.

Vuber Core cartridge & Pulse battery

Most refillable vape cartridges have two main drawbacks; the difficulty of actually refiling the cart and the use of metal heating coils and cotton or synthetic fiber "wicks." The first issue causes many users immense frustration, particularly when product is wasted during filling, which often happens because the "center post" in most carts obstructs the chamber. This can also cause obstruct airflow and damage the heating mechanism if oil gets inside that center post. The use of fiber wicking and coils often imparts harsh, unpleasant "burnt" flavors to the vapor, undermining the desired flavor profile and potentially harming the health of the consumer.

The Vuber Core cartridge addresses both of these issues with an open cart design that eliminates the center post and the wicks and coils. The atomizer instead uses porous glass filtration and flash heating to create a clean, flavorful vapor free of any irritants or contaminants.

But what about those prefillled carts you buy from your favorite extractor? Some of those may still have traditional wicking. This is where the Vuber Pulse battery comes in with its "never burn" heating system, that au-

tomatically adjusts the battery output to match the resistance of the cart without overheating. It can be used with any 510 thread cartridge, making it as versatile as a traditional Ego style batter, but with automatic heat control that will preserve your flavor no matter what you attach to it.

VAPE "PENS"

Portable "vape pen" vaporizers have become ubiquitous, particularly in decriminalized states like California, where you can find adults of all ages puffing at discrete, handheld devices just about anywhere. As with other types of vaporizers, there's a wide array of different functional and stylistic options, but only a handful of fundamental approaches to vaporizing cannabis.

As with most cultural and technological developments in cannabis, the terminology isn't precise, and many people lump any pocket-sized vaporizer into the "pen" category, which is what we've done in this chapter. Some people further distinguish between devices roughly the shape and size of a cigarette and slightly larger devices, but the basic technology is the same: A small battery fitted to some kind of atomizer, which either heats up at the push of a button or in response to inhalation. These devices are also sometimes called "dab pens" because they're largely used to consume concentrates, which some people refer to using the catchall "dabs."

When it comes to "pen"-style vaporizers, there are a few basic characteristics —most devices will check off at least two of these boxes:

- Prefilled or reloadable
- Rechargeable or disposable
- Conduction or convection
- Button or breath activated

When people first started using dab pens, they were generally inexpensive combinations of a small, cylindrical battery pack (roughly the size of a roll of breath mints) and a small atomizer (a heating element that produces vapor) contained in a glass dome — roughly the size of a pinball. The atomizer dome was attached to the battery's threaded contact point, the button on the battery heated the atomizer coils and the material on it would vaporize through conduction, collecting inside the glass dome where it was inhaled through a mouthpiece fitted into the top. It was crude, and they broke all the time — the heating element and the glass part — but they were the standard until companies started really doing R&D around handheld concentrate vaporizers.

While the core principle of an atomizer that vaporizes through conduction is still central to most handheld vape pens, the materials and construction have improved and the housing has grown more durable. There used to be synthetic fabric "wicks" inside the heating coils, adding unpleasant tastes to the vapor. With most new atomizers for concentrate, the coils have either

been removed from the material area or the wicking has been replaced by ceramic or quartz rods. And those that still used glass pieces offer them in more elaborate styles; there are now water percolator attachments and almost any other smoking accessory one could imagine fitted specifically for the threaded contract points and atomizer sizes of vape pens.

REFILLABLE DAB PENS

Dank Fung Connoisseur

Some refillable dab pens use pro-prietary connectors, but the Dank Fung Connoisseur offers compact, durable, refillable vaporizers with a battery base threaded to also ac-cept prefilled cartridges; the man-ufacturers claim that it will heat them more efficiently than smaller batteries, but your mileage may

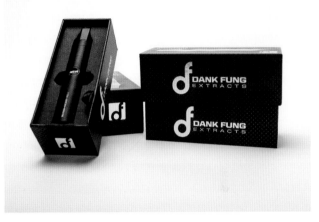

vary. What you definitely will notice if you're used to the old-school coil atomizers is the flavor difference between that and an all-ceramic dish atomizer, which removes all the unpleasant fla-vors of fabric wicks and/or low-grade coils, leaving only the even, more or less neutral flavor profile of ceramic conduction heating.

The Connoisseur isn't the cheapest device of its kind, but with a price tag under $100 (gen-erally retailing for about $90) it's a fairly accessible option for those seeking something a bit more substantial than a generic battery. The wider and deeper than average atomizer dish al-lows for easier loading and can handle any kind of concentrate, including shatter, distillate, and rosin. Its single-temperature, one-button interface may appeal more to new dab pen users than experienced ones, but the unique battery system will prove useful to anyone: Most vape pen batteries avoid overheating by cutting off the power after 10 seconds of continuous heating, but the Connoisseur "pulses" the power, which allows for less restricted use and more vapor production, and keeps the device from getting too hot. Despite this difference, the battery still uses the standard 5-click locking mechanism.

The Executive model from Dank Fung offers a more stylish aesthetic, with a pen-cap housing similar to the Dopen but coated in 24-karat rose gold. A quartz-rod atomizer and clear-glass vapor chamber, along with three temperature settings, provide flavorful vapor and quick, intuitive temperature customization. These extra features come with a price tag — the Executive retails for about $140 — but for those seeking a fashion forward yet discrete, unit with just enough functionality, this is a solid option.

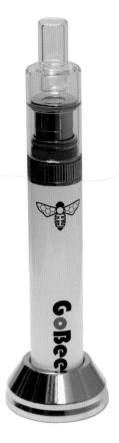

GoBee and GoBee Plus

Bee-Nail is already associated with its namesake e-nail, so it's no real surprise that the company also branched out into portable concentrate vaporizers. Those familiar with the company's stationary dabbing gear will enjoy the same reliability and precision, albeit in a slightly less powerful but portable package.

The GoBee series is also a good choice for those seeking a sturdy device that can take a beating without affecting the functionality; for $80 to $100 or so (depending on the particular model selected) the GoBee will soldier on through accidental falls and impacts without harming its performance. It is a bit heavy given that it's larger in size and thicker than the average battery — but whatever it comes into contact with in the event of a drop is probably in more danger than it is. For some users, this hefty weight will be a downside, but for those who like a more substantial unit with an extended battery life (up to 5 days on a single charge) the GoBee is perfect.

The only breakable part on the device is the glass mouthpiece, but this concession to flavor at the cost of durability pays off, particularly in concert with the quartz coil atomizer and a shorter-than-usual vapor path, creating a perfect device for enjoying big, dense clouds of flavorful vapor on the go. And if durability is an overriding concern, the GoBee Plus offers an unbreakable titanium mouthpiece. The oddest feature of the GoBee is the button placement, which is found at the base of the battery rather than on the side. It's a little weird, but doesn't meaningfully undermine the usability.

DISPOSABLE OIL CARTRIDGES | CONCENTRATE ONLY

Some consumers, particularly connoisseurs of top-shelf concentrates, prefer concentrate vaporizers that allow them to consume the same products they dab, but not everyone has the time or desire to deal with loading, cleaning, and reloading chambers and heating elements — they just want to puff on the fly wherever they are. This desire for a small, simple option for concentrate consumption has led to the widespread embrace of disposable cartridge-based "pen" vaporizers.

These "carts" come filled with cannabis concentrate, which is sometimes cut with food-grade fillers like propylene glycol or vegetable glycerin, but most users prefer the pure concentrate variety, now often filled with distillate. Most brands offer a package that includes a battery attachment, but the threading on batteries and cartridges, regardless of cartridge volume or battery voltage, are more or less universal. There are certain proprietary attachments and

systems, but the majority will be interchangeable, meaning you can purchase a durable battery you like and use it to heat any cartridge. Most serious concentrate consumers find uses for both profiled and refillable pens.

In fact, one of the most popular systems — the Pax Era — has completely proprietary carts and attachments. So you can't use brands that aren't approved by Pax on the Era, and you can't use the Era carts on any other battery base — think of it like the "walled garden" Apple created on the iPhone; some people like that extra layer of curation and simplicity, others want the freedom to use any app they want. There are people who love iPhones and those who prefer Android phones, and those same considerations are a big part of what will decide if you prefer a "proprietary" cart system or an "open source" one. That said, all the examples below are actually interchangeable, so sometimes it's just a matter of aesthetics or personal preference for the contents of the carts.

A NOTE ON BATTERIES, OR WHY YOUR BATTERY JUST "STOPPED WORKING"

It's no coincidence that most batteries and cartridges have compatible connection points — the vast majority of vape pens use the same core battery technology. That also means the function and features are roughly the same across most makes and models, and one nearly universal feature is the 5-click battery lock/unlock feature; it's also a common source of frustration for new battery owners who aren't always aware of it.

By clicking the power/heat activator button five times in rapid succession, you can either lock or unlock it. When the button is locked, pressing it won't activate the atomizer, which is great if the pen is in your pocket and you aren't pushing the button on purpose. Accidental activation could result in painful burns or pose a fire hazard, making the lock function practical. But just as the vape function on the battery can be triggered inadvertently, so can the locking mechanism meant to prevent that from happening. It's a common enough occurrence for new battery owners; they pop the pen in their pocket without locking it — because they don't even know they can lock it — and when they pull it out, it's "broken." If your battery isn't working, always check and make sure it isn't just locked.

Dopen

The Dopen isn't just a battery; it's a stylish pen with some extra functionality built in and a flip cover that protects the charging port. It also has magnetic connecting pieces that allow you to discretely take off the top to show just the tip of the mouthpiece, not the cartridge. For about $40 retail you get the Dopen battery, which is compatible with all 510 thread prefilled cartridges, and comes with a USB charger. The unit is especially discrete; it comes housed in what really looks like a pen, complete with a cap fitted with a shirt clip. It also offers three temperature settings — low, medium, and high — 1.8 volts, 2.6 volts, and 3.4 volts respectively. These settings are represented by a blue, green, and yellow light, making it easy to adjust on the fly. Limited-edition versions are created with different prints that make these effective pens worth the upgrade.

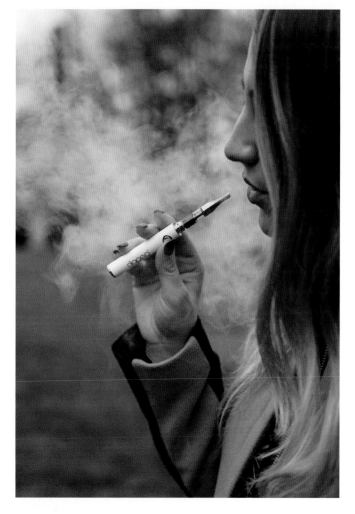

We've provided some examples of cartridge-based vaporizers, but many consumers purchase a battery separately and buy cartridges from whatever brand they prefer. There are some advantages to proprietary cartridge systems, but most people prefer the ability to screw on any cartridge they want. A standard, threaded Ego-style vaporizer battery should accommodate most cartridges — almost all extractors fill the same kind of cart.

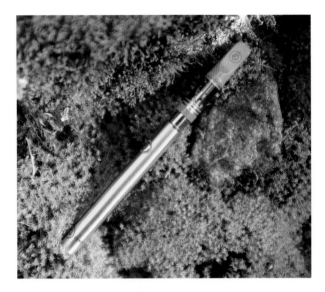

Zensi Pen Cartridges

The Zensi Pen is an easy-to-use, fixed-voltage battery with an attractive metallic exterior and a smooth, ergonomic push button placed nearly flush with the unit. That said, if you already own a threaded battery base for cartridge vaping, you can still attach Zensi Cartridges, which are available in three strain-specific styles: "Tranquil & Relaxing" Indica, "Bright & Bold" Sativa, and "Sweet & Balanced" Hybrid. They also offer CBD distillate cartridges, which are perfect for those seeking immediate relief from inflammation and other CBD-responsive ailments.

Unlike many cartridge manufacturers, the founders of Zensi cultivated cannabis for two decades before branching out into concentrates. That well-developed understanding of the plant shows in the potent, flavorful oils they produce using popular strains like Girl Scout Cookies and Gorilla Glue #4. There are so many cartridges to choose from, but Zensi is definitely on the list of ones you must try.

Outer Galactic Vapes™
Oil Pen

Outer Galactic is best known for their award winning chocolates, which have a distinctly cosmic appearance inspired by nebulae. But the company also produces out of this world vape pens, which come with pre-filled distillate cartridges attached. The design is simple but the battery base is perfect for those seeking the lowest profile and simplest

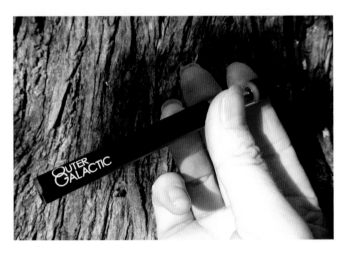

function; it's matte black, roughly the shape and length of a pen or a king size cigarette, and it's draw activated, meaning it heats up automatically when you hit it; no button required and no chance of it accidentally heating up in your pocket.

The oil inside the cartridges is especially flavorful, and while the pens are not strain specific, the fresh, natural flavor of the vapor is much more akin to taking a puff from a joint than many of the fruit and candy flavors offered by other distillate manufacturers. On balance, the Outer Galactic is a perfect option for vapers seeking out a clean, simple expression of cannabis in a no-fuss, low-maintenance package.

Avitas CCELL CO$_2$ cartridge

Unlike many cartridges that use distillate, Avitas carts are filled with full-spectrum CO$_2$ oil. The terpene profile has been preserved, not isolated and re-added or formulated from scratch, and many consumers find they prefer the effects of a full-spectrum oil. This on its own is a reason to try the Avitas CCell CO$_2$ carts.

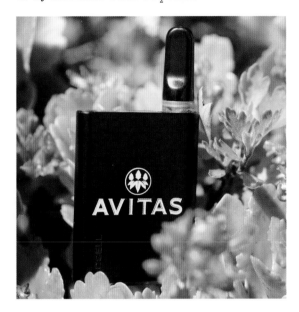

The flavor of the CCell carts is superior to those that use cotton fiber and other wicking mechanisms because it relies on porous ceramic. This proprietary technology creates a smoother flavor, eliminating the unpleasant burnt flavor associated with low-grade carts.

A full kit includes the CCell battery base, which can hold a charge for up to a week without recharging. Because of its slender styling, it can easily fit in a back pocket, making it ideal for those with an active lifestyle who spend time outdoors away from outlets.

And if you own a Pax Era, you can purchase Avitas full-spectrum CO$_2$ oil in a Pax-compatible cart — they're Pax approved, if that's your thing. Regardless of how you consume it, Avitas oil offers a unique option in a market largely glutted with distillate carts.

It's hard to overstate how ubiquitous oil pens are becoming, particularly among frequent air travelers, who've collectively deemed them the gold standard for inconspicuous transportation and use, even when flying internationally. That popularity is driving an intense demand for what usually goes inside those cartridges — CO$_2$ concentrate or cannabis distillate.

Dank Fung

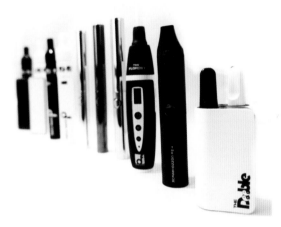

As both a producer and a patient in the state of Connecticut, Daniel Fung was eager to try vaporizers when they first started to appear on the market, but his enthusiasm was dampened by his experiences with the first generation of devices. He wasn't tasting the flavor of the terpenes, and wanted more precise control over the temperature throughout the smoking experience. So he did what any clever entrepreneur would do – he researched the technology and started to build and design his own.

After an exhaustive 6-month study of many different styles and types of heater technologies, he built three different vape pen prototypes, and conducted trials with industry peers. After testing the different models, he started to realize that low temperature vaporization not only eliminates the inhalation of carcinogens, but it also allows users to appreciate the full floral taste of the products.

"As extraction artists by trade, we design all of our products to maximize terpene appreciation and enjoyment," said Fung. "We use terpene appreciation as a guiding hallmark in how we develop all of our products."

In 2016, Dank Fung started operations in Oregon, but as sales grew it needed to scale up warehousing and fulfillment to accommodate demand. In 2017 the company moved its headquarters to California, where it was officially incorporated. By the summer of 2017, the company was getting positive press for its products, including a top spot in the High Times Annual Vape Pen Review for its for its Executive 24K gold plated Vape Pen. That award led to a strong uptick in sales, and plenty of interest from other publications that wanted to do product reviews.

Dank Fung's signature line of concentrate vape pens have been specially designed to enjoy a one-of-a-kind terpene experience. The company's unique, luxury vape pens feature lower heating temps and wickless, ceramic, sub ohm atomizers that emphasize freshness and vapor cloud production, as well as longer life between refills.

"I came to realize that just as America is a melting pot of many cultures, there are many different lifestyles of marijuana consumers in existence," said Fung. "So instead of just calling my vape pens, DFE vape pen 1.0, 2.0, 3.0., I named them as if I was designing them for a particular person's lifestyle."

The Executive is for the business person that still likes to unwind after a long day's work reaching for marijuana instead of a beer. The Florist is a flower only vaping device, so it was named after an occupation that appreciates the flower first and foremost.

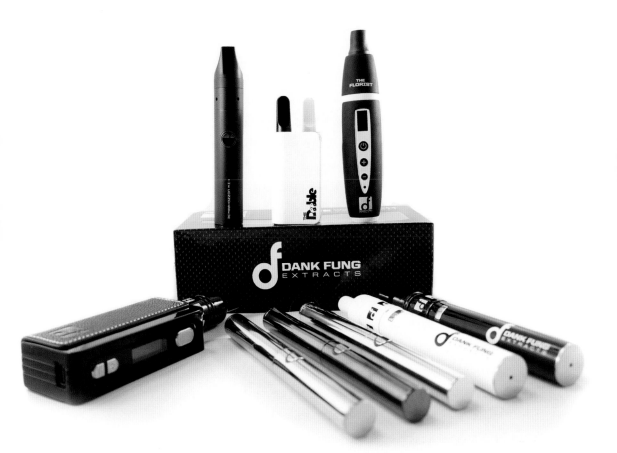

Disorderly Conduction

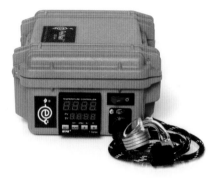

When the first generation of e-nails hit the market in 2013, the early models were somewhat crude, and also presented safety hazards, due to the cheap materials used and unsafe electrical wiring. Disorderly Conduction was founded in Southern California in 2014 with the express mission of providing a safe, effective, and stylish electronic nail to the growing community of cannabis concentrate connoisseurs.

Since e-nails maintain high temperatures for extended periods of time, the design details and manufacturing technique really does matter, and Disorderly Conduction knew that the safety of its devices was a principal concern. So from the beginning, the company ensured that all of the wiring for its production was done in-house by an experienced electrician, using high-quality materials and craftsmanship to ensure that customers have the safest and most enjoyable dabbing experience possible.

Its flagship concept, The PeliNail, is a combination of two of the most highly sought after products in the industry – top of the line American made Pelican Cases, and reliable, easy to use, safe and accurate e-nails.

How does an e-nail work, you ask?

The PeliNail is powered by a digitally controlled heating unit that is plugged into a power supply, and a digital display allows the user to set a desired temperature. Extending from the heating unit is a Kevlar cord, or "whip", with a metal coil attached to the end. Electronically generated heat is transferred from the heating unit, through the whip, to the coil. The metal coil is sized to fit specific titanium or quartz domeless nails, and the heat from the coil transfers to the dish of the domeless nail, bringing the dabbing surface to the user's exact desired temperature.

There are six different options available for coil sizes, ranging from 16mm up to 30mm, including a "flat" version as well. This ensures that no matter which domeless nail is in use – titanium or quartz – Disorderly Conduction has the perfect coil option in stock.

In addition to providing the safest, most reliable e-nails in the industry, Disorderly Conduction has also been responsive to its customers' requests for new product designs.

When the demand grew for smaller, more discreet and easy to transport PeliNails, the company designed the Micro PeliNail 1030. At just 7.5 inches long, and just under 4 inches wide, the Micro PeliNail puts the full power of its larger units right into the palm of your hand. The case itself is water-resistant, dustproof, and crushproof. There are currently four colors available, as well as a clear version that features a choice of four colored inserts and shows off the expert wiring that the company takes pride in.

To address the growing need for a mobile dab rig, Disorderly Conduction developed a solution with its DC Portable Battery Pack. When e-nails were first introduced, users needed to be near a power outlet to supply the proper amount of power that the average e-nail draws. This seemed like a needless limitation, so the company developed the DC Portable Battery Pack so users could take their dab sessions on the road. A 2-hour charge time gives users a comparable constant runtime of 2-3 hours anywhere that their adventures may take them. Beach dabs, anyone?

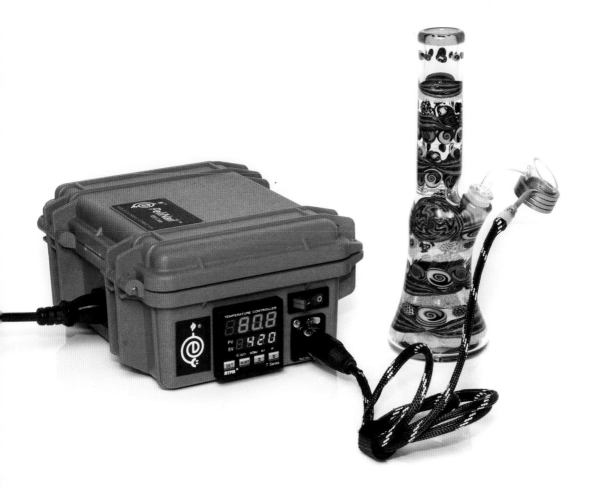

Mendo Breath shatter by Pissing Excellence
Photo: Fred Morlege

CHAPTER 3

BHO:
Butane Hash Oil — Shatter, Wax, Sauce, and Beyond

The impact of solvent extraction on the cannabis industry has been nothing short of revolutionary, and if any single solvent can be credited with taking trim from *Trash to Stash* in terms of market value, it's butane — the undisputed favorite for solvent extraction.

There are several factors behind butane's popularity. In a nutshell, it's the cheapest, most efficient solvent and offers the most desirable final product. Additionally, where other methods concentrate carcinogenic tars, chlorophyll, and microbial contaminants from the source material, butane extraction strips away plant waxes and eliminates or neutralizes most fungi, bacteria, mold, and other impurities.

While there are consumers who prefer "classically extracted" full-spectrum hash or rosin, a growing number of people prefer butane hash oil (BHO) — people love it and will pay top dollar for it if it's made well. The golden translucence of a properly purged shatter quite different from the earthy opacity of a water or dry-sift hash. The efficient isolation of terpenes from chlorophyll and plant lipids offers a crystal clear expression of a plant's flavor profile, one that's almost impossible to replicate by smoking or vaping raw buds.

When it comes to potency, most BHO contains upward of 75% THC, with many brands consistently testing in the mid-80s. That's well over the average potency of high-grade raw cannabis, which generally tests somewhere between 18 and 20% THC.

TERP TIME

Processors love butane because it's cheap, easy to find and buy, the processing equipment needed isn't prohibitively expensive, and it offers the highest extraction efficiency. But what really sets the final product apart is the terpene profile. Butane extraction is a cold process, which preserves the highly prized but incredibly delicate terpenes and aromatic molecules.

As covered in a previous chapter, terpenes are the molecular building blocks of flavor and smell found in all organic material. Where most fruits or flowers produce a fairly predictable terpene profile (smelling roughly the same plant to plant), in the case of cannabis, there is a practically limitless spectrum of distinct terpene profiles. With cannabis plants, terpenes don't just form the flavor: they also inform the effects of the final product.

There's an expanding array of styles when it comes to BHO, ranging from standard waxes and shatters to live resin and crystalline terp sauce. Although the initial extraction process is the same, differences in the purge process (explanation below) create physical characteristics that are more or less desirable, depending on the end goal and target market.

Some of the more advanced methods of BHO production require additional labor to achieve results, but these products will also generally command a much higher price than basic extractions.

Bottom line, for extractors looking to maximize the flavor, potency, and value of their harvest while removing practically all vegetative material and carcinogenic impurities, butane extraction could be the way to go. It's the most popular chemical extraction process for a reason.

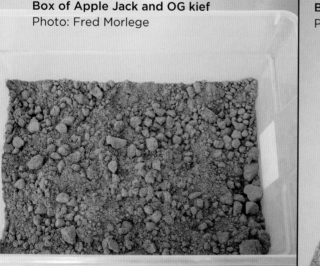

Box of Apple Jack and OG kief
Photo: Fred Morlege

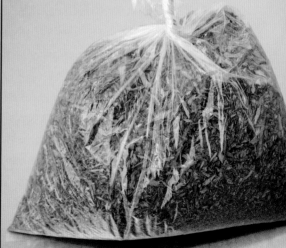

Bag of trim at Pissing Excellence
Photo: Fred Morlege

BLASTING BASICS

HOW IT WORKS

The ultimate goal of all concentrate extraction is the same: Separate the resin glands from the buds. What makes solvent extraction different from other methods is the precision with which it targets the desirable elements — cannabinoids and terpenes, both of which are contained within the resin glands, also called trichomes.

Those macro-lens super close-ups of cannabis plants featured in magazines? Those are showcasing the trichomes — the little translucent mushrooms clinging to the buds, what many people used to call "crystals."

Instead of relying on physical agitation to remove the glands, butane extraction dissolves them, creating a "resin" — the removed cannabinoids and terpenes and the liquid solvent. Because its boiling point is so low, much of the residual butane will evaporate at room temperature, but some will still be trapped inside the resin. At that point, the use of a vacuum oven will be required to remove the residual solvent and determine the style of BHO created.

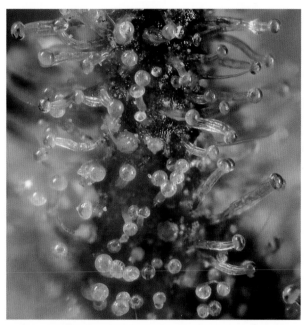

Calyx - Relic Seeds Photo by Professor P. / Dynasty Genetics

Regardless of which style of BHO you're planning to produce or which method you intend to use, the fundamentals of the initial process are always the same; "run" butane through raw cannabis buds to dissolve the cannabinoids, terpenes, and other active ingredients from the plant matter, then evaporate the solvent. What's left behind is highly concentrated resin with trace amounts of solvent that still need to be purged. Depending on the process used for the purge and the physical qualities of your plant matter and resulting resin, your end product could look like any of the styles listed we explore in this book.

There are two primary methods for handling this process — open blasting and closed-loop extraction — but before choosing which is ideal, it's crucial to understand and account for the substantial hazards associated with both approaches.

SAFETY WARNING

Butane is highly flammable, and the most basic BHO extraction method — open blasting — creates substantial risk for explosions and fires if serious precautions are not taken. If performed incorrectly, it doesn't just place the extractor at risk; it endangers everyone nearby. There's no shortage of tragic stories about failed BHO labs that turned into deadly explosions and fires.

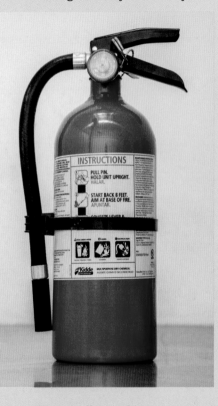

If a person were to try the most popular extraction method, he or she would select butane extraction. But it can't be stressed enough, if they wanted to pick the most dangerous method of concentrate extraction, he or she would still end up with butane extraction — it cannot be overstated how volatile this process is.

This isn't just an ethical consideration; in addition to the physical risks, many municipalities view BHO production with the same jaundiced eye as narcotics manufacturing, meaning that the legal consequences can be severe — and they aren't likely to show leniency to violators who also hurt or kill somebody when their "lab" explodes.

Technically speaking, anyone with a tube, some low-grade trim, and a few cans of butane can extract high-grade BHO. Practically speaking, it's an industrial process that should only be performed by trained professionals under controlled conditions. To safely extract with butane, the process must be performed in a specialized room fitted with explosion-proof electrical components, called "Class 1, Division 1" components. BHO production requires much more than a "well-ventilated room"; even using a lab hood, which intuitively seems like a solution, will not ensure a safe environment.

For all these reasons, everyone involved in *Beyond Buds: Next Generation* adamantly advises against any attempt to extract BHO outside a legally permitted laboratory.

GO BIG OR DON'T GO

Avoid using canned butane, regardless of can size or alleged purity — ignore labels claiming "research grade" contents or touting numerous degrees of filtration: ALL cans of butane contain impurities. These include various machine oils used as lubricants for the machinery used to fill the cans, which also serve as rust protectant for the can linings and as propelling agents that prevent clogging. Additionally, most canned butane contains mercaptans, which give the otherwise odorless gas a strong smell for leak detection purposes. These chemicals make up what has been called "mystery oil," because they are part of

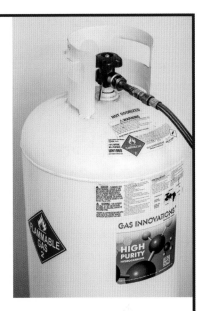

the butane production process that does not have to be disclosed and are listed in the ingredients as "one percent other."

Closed-loop extractors can be used to purify cheap butane and remove the mystery oil by running the solvent through the machine without plant material. That said, there's no real cost benefit to doing this — it's just extra work — so use "laboratory grade" 99.5% pure or 99.9% pure butane, called instrument n-butane, from one of the major national suppliers. A tank the size of a typical BBQ grill tank can be used to extract roughly 20 pounds of cannabis. Generally, 5 pounds of solvent per pound of starting material or 1 can per oz.

WHAT MAKES BUTANE SO EXPLOSIVE?

Butane has an exceptionally low boiling point — just under the temperature at which water freezes. For that reason, it takes the form of a gas at room temperature, but it's a gas that's heavier than air. So instead of diffusing into the air or "off-gassing," it sinks to the floor, pooling and flowing as it slowly evaporates unless it finds a source of ignition: A pilot light or hot-water heater, or even just a tiny, invisible spark of normally harmless static electricity is all that is needed to create an explosion with potentially devastating consequences.

It really should go without saying, but never smoke or use a cell phone around butane extraction equipment. Static electricity causes more BHO fires than smoking: Avoid wool and synthetic fabric to minimize that risk. Cotton fabrics like denim, which have static control, can help limit injuries during a flash fire. That said, there is no substitute for a laboratory-grade fireproof suit.

BUTANE EXTRACTION IS DANGEROUS — BHO CONSUMPTION IS NOT

There's a lot of mixed information (and misinformation) when it comes to the safety of the end product of butane extraction, specifically relating to the potential danger of consuming trace amounts of "residual solvent."

Butane is used in food-processing and food-flavoring production, so you're probably already consuming residual butane regularly. Thankfully, it's pretty safe. According to research cited by the CDC, even prolonged exposure to 10,000 ppm of butane for 10 minutes "may lead to drowsiness, but does not appear to cause systemic effects."[1] In Berkeley, California — home of the most stringent cap on residual solvents in BHO — the limit on total combined residuals is 400 ppm, and in Colorado it's 500 ppm.

From a consumer standpoint, if the presence of residuals can be detected using any of the five senses, then the levels are unacceptably high; the taste threshold for butane is 300 ppm, so today's market is full of professional extractors who consistently test below that. That said, the only sure-fire way to know the ppm level is a lab test. When extracting for a regulated market like California, testing is the law.

Of course, terpenes are extracted along with cannabinoids, and since terpenes are natural solvents, the same purge process that targets residuals will also reduce the final terpene content. The dance between hitting target ppm levels — officially mandated or otherwise — and preserving the valuable terpene profile is one performed by every extractor. That's the part of the process that is more art than science.

OPEN BLASTING: HOW IT WORKS AND WHY NOVICES SHOULD NOT DO IT

Open blasting doesn't reuse butane, which makes it inefficient; it also makes it expensive. On top of that, it's a more dangerous process. There are steps you can take to minimize and mitigate the risks involved, but there's really no way to fully ensure safety when open blasting. Doing it outdoors can reduce the potential for a fire, but an explosion is an explosion and it's always dangerous.

Unless you're an experienced professional, do not use this method of extraction. Here is a quick overview of how open blasting works when performed safely and under the right conditions:

---

[1]G. Clayton and F. Clayton, eds., *Patty's Industrial Hygiene and Toxicology*, 3rd rev. ed. (New York: Wiley & Sons, 1981), accessed via "Occupational Safety and Health Guidelines for n-Butane," U.S. Department of Health and Human Services, https://www.cdc.gov/niosh/docs/81-123/pdfs/0068.pdf

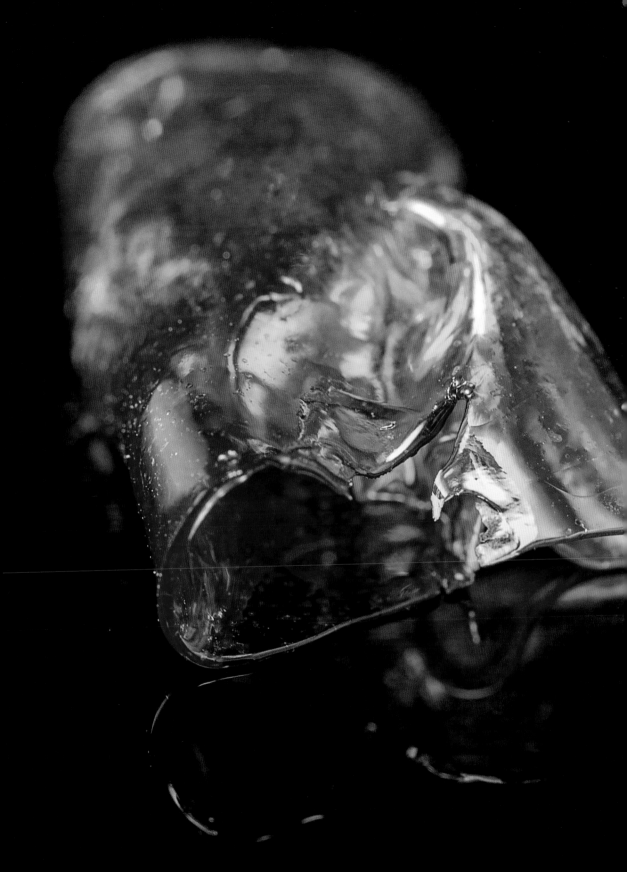

BHO Concentrate Photo by Professor P / Dynasty Genetics

MATERIALS NEEDED

- Butane canisters (one canister per ounce) w/filling adapter if needed
- Thick-gauge, 2"-wide, 25"-long Pyrex glass or stainless steel extraction tubes (stainless steel is stronger; Pyrex makes it easier to see what's going on inside the tube)
- Coffee filters (unbleached)
- Source plant material (trichome-rich, fresh-cured, cleaned of debris, chopped up)
- Large Pyrex casserole dishes for catching trays for solution
- Parchment paper
- Safety glasses
- Organic vapor-rated gas mask
- Large fan
- Flame- and cold-resistant gloves
- Implements: dishes, trays, scrapers, jars
- Powderless latex gloves
- Laser thermometer
- Chemical fire extinguisher
- Fireproof suit

PROCESS

The physical process of open blasting is simple: Fill the tube with cannabis, run the solvent through the tube, and purge the extracted resin. Depending on the specific tube setup you use, some steps may be slightly different, but the basics are the same.

1. Attach the coffee filters to the bottom of the tube. Depending on the tube you're using, it may have a "salt shaker" cap with several holes on the bottom. You can affix the filter over this cap or place it inside. Just make sure it's fully covering the bottom so plant material doesn't get into your resin.
2. Pack the tube with ground buds and/or trim using a wooden dowel. Don't overpack the tube, particularly a glass tube, which can shatter under pressure if packed too tightly.
3. Position the pyrex dish so it can collect the resin from the tube and position the fan so it pushes gas away from the extraction site.
4. Orient the tube vertically over the dish with the filtered end down and the discharge cap end up. Some tubes will have a top cap with a hole fitted for your butane canister tip, otherwise, use a filling adapter.
5. Discharge individual canisters into the tube and allow the pressurized butane liquid (now rich with cannabinoids and terpenes) to collect in the dish.

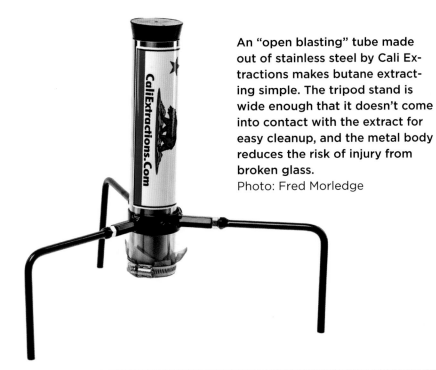

An "open blasting" tube made out of stainless steel by Cali Extractions makes butane extracting simple. The tripod stand is wide enough that it doesn't come into contact with the extract for easy cleanup, and the metal body reduces the risk of injury from broken glass.
Photo: Fred Morledge

SAFETY NOTE

Because of the physical characteristics of butane, the tube will get incredibly cold during the extraction process. Gloves should be worn for skin protection. Stainless steel, for this reason, is ideal — it won't shatter, whereas moisture from the air can collect on a glass tube, freezing and breaking it. The Pyrex tray of liquid solution will also get very cold.

6. Collect the resin from the dish and purge it. Ultimately, regardless of extraction method, the only reliable and safe way to purge the product is to use a vacuum oven.

DON'T USE A HOT PLATE

Those news stories about people blowing up their home or apartment trying to extract BHO? Many of those explosions happened because somebody was trying to purge resin on a hot plate or using a double boiler: DO NOT USE THOSE METHODS TO PURGE BHO. There is no safe way to purge using a hot plate, no matter how many fans or exhaust hoods you employ. Don't perform solvent extraction unless you're ready to invest in a vacuum oven for a professional purge.

Extractor Depot closed loop extractor
extracting live resin at Pissing Excellence
Photo: Fred Morlege

CLOSED-LOOP EXTRACTION: HOW IT WORKS

As we delve into the procedural particulars of solvent extraction, it's important to keep these basic principles in mind to avoid getting bogged down in technical details: Extract as cold and as quickly as possible, then purge slowly, using the lowest heat possible. If you keep that basic idea at the forefront of your process, you'll already be well on your way.

SOLVENT EXTRACTION — QUICK & COLD: Minimize the contact time during a solvent pass. Longer passes will increase yields, but as always, those higher yields come from the inclusion of less desirable components like lipids and waxes. If your end goal is to produce a flavorful wax, shatter, or sugar, you need to keep the passes quick and cold. If you're producing "crude" oil for further distillation, then it might make sense to prioritize yield over quality, but just remember: the quicker and colder, the cleaner, and better the end result.

PURGING BHO — SLOW & LOW: There's no need to rush when it comes to your purge process, and doing so can be dangerous to you and damaging to your end product. We recommend allowing your freshly extracted BHO to off-gas at regular atmospheric pressure / room temperature for 24 hours before placing it in a vacuum oven. When you do get to the vacuum oven stage, remember how pressure affects heat — the reason vacuum ovens are used in the first place. At higher atmospheric pressure, the boiling point of solvents are reduced, allowing for effective removal without compromising color or flavor with high heat. Think of it like jumping on the moon; your jumping ability hasn't changed, but the reduced gravity means you can jump roughly ten feet in the air. Make sure you're taking time to slowly purge — 72 hours or more — at a temperature no higher than 120°F.

In the early days of butane extraction, creating a closed-loop system required a great deal of research and usually a bit of tinkering. Now there are several reputable companies that produce relatively affordable commercial extraction systems tailored specifically to the needs of solvent extractors working with cannabis. Whether you construct your own system from scratch or purchase a prefabricated unit, the basic components are roughly the same.

BASIC COMPONENTS

All butane extraction systems contain some common elements, although there are many variations on the theme.

Butane reservoir — the butane tank holds the liquid butane, the solvent for the extraction

Trim tube — a stainless steel cylinder that is packed with trim

Evaporation chamber — the tank used to catch and hold the raw solution of butane and the extracted cannabinoids, waxes, etc.; here the solvent is separated from the oil again

Vacuum pump — a butane-proof, high-quality, high-speed pump used to create the vacuum or pressure needed to use the extractor

Recovery pump — used in many systems to accelerate the process of returning recycled butane to the reservoir

Vacuum oven — an industrial oven that pairs with a pump to create a vacuum inside, used to purge BHO of residual solvent

Gas detectors — to warn of any potential leaks or hazards

MATERIALS NEEDED

- N-butane tanks
- Butane closed-loop extractor with recapture
- Filters (Whatman lab-grade, medium and slow filters)
- Source plant material (freshly dried and cured, trichome-rich)
- Oil-less refrigeration recovery pump (master vapor)
- Vacuum oven
- Multistage vacuum pump for oven and closed-loop system (8 or higher CFM)
- Safety glasses
- Gas mask
- Cold-resistant lab gloves
- Implements: dishes, trays, scrapers, jars
- Laser thermometer
- Chemical fire extinguisher
- Fireproof suit

PROCESS

The key to getting a good result from closed-loop extraction is fast, cold solvent passes, but it's also important to ensure proper moisture levels in the material — it should either be very dry or very cold. Typical buds purchased at a dispensary or retail outlet contain roughly 6%–8% water by dry weight. The use of desiccants is a common approach to getting the material dry and will prevent the terpene loss incurred by methods that involve heating: Many terpenes are volatilized at low temperatures, meaning that a rushed drying process could reduce the quality of the final product.

Some extractors freeze the material to keep the moisture in a solid form rather than drying it — this technique is covered in the "Live Resin" chapter.

Once appropriate material is secured, clean all parts of the extraction system with denatured alcohol; some gaskets can be wiped clean using olive oil.

Add 1 pound of trim and/or buds to the tube on the top of the chamber. Pack it with a wooden dowel, but not too tightly.

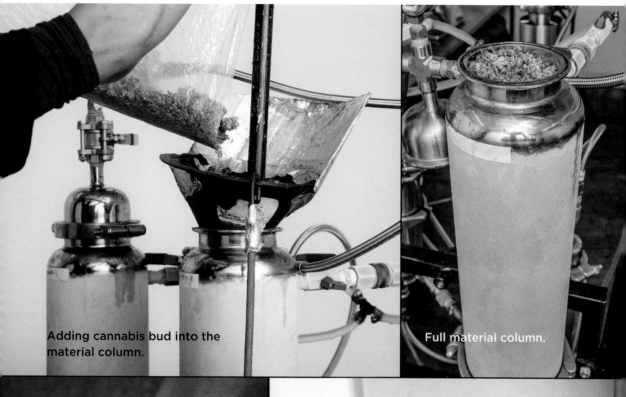

Adding cannabis bud into the material column.

Full material column.

Filter

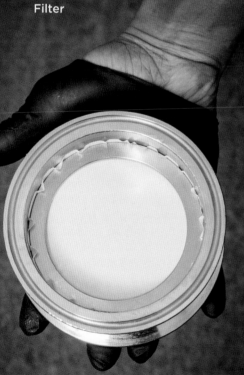

Adding the filter to the material column. Pissing Excellence
Photo: Fred Morlege

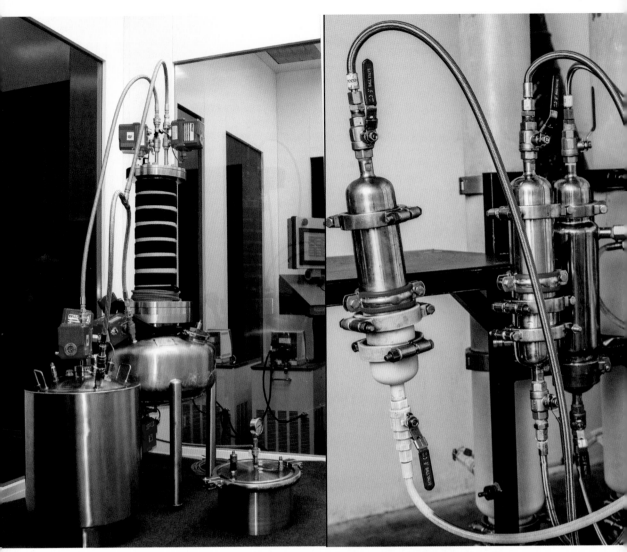

A Tamisium extractor in a lab setting

Carbon filters, Pissing Excellence
Photo: Fred Morlege

Tamisium Inc. manufactures botanical and herbal extractors. Tamisium's closed passive extractor design solves closed loop extractor issues that continue to challenge extractors across the industry. Their revolutionary extractors allow digital tracking of inventory beginning with where the material is sourced to its final sale to an end consumer.

This enables extraction companies to be more efficient and states to manage inventory across the entire distribution chain: Tax revenue can be predicted and the benefits of various products can be shown along with demand, supply, cost and consumer demographics.

The extraction lab is the point of production and the first place the product can be weighed and measured for standardized dosing. As the industry evolves, the extraction labs with the ability to formulate repeat and track their products will be the most successful.

Extracted oil in the sight glass
material column, Pissing Excellence
Photo: Fred Morlege

Install filters. Assemble collection vessel, viewing chamber, valves, packed trim tube, and shower head ball cap. Use the vacuum pump to pull the entire system down to a full vacuum (-20–30 mm Hg) in the system. This vacuum will help identify any leaks in the system before it's used. It also pulls any remaining water out of the system and helps pull the butane out of its reservoir, through the plant matter, and into the evaporation chamber.

Recapture extractors run in a big loop, with the ability of the operator to interrupt the circuit and send the solvent into a frozen recovery tank.

Check all connections. Make sure the clamps are really tight and the system is truly closed.

After the system is tested for leaks, warm up the butane reservoir with a hot water bath to give it some pressure, attach it to the system, and slowly open the butane tank valve. The liquid solvent will rush through the tubes and begin filling up the trim tube. A manual butterfly valve sends the solution in the tube through the filters, past the viewing vessel, to pool in the collection reservoir.

At first, the system yields high-end white, yellow, amber, or clear extract. The longer the system runs, the more cannabinoids are yielded, but the extract also becomes darker and lower quality from plant waxes and other oil solubles. Remember — quicker, colder, cleaner; quicker passes will extract less of the undesirable elements, like plant lipids and waxes, producing a slightly lower yield but also a cleaner, more attractive product.

Depending on the pump, a one-pound extractor takes about half an hour to run a barbecue-sized tank of butane through three times. Check the pressure gauges regularly.

WINTERIZING

Winterizing is a process that removes inert plant solids from the liquid solution to increase "stability," giving the end product a firmer "shatter" consistency rather than a sappy, goopy, or waxy one. This isn't a strictly necessary step, and there are certain popular BHO styles that rely on the retention of some fats and waxes to achieve certain textures. That said, there is conclusive evidence that the long-term inhalation of those plant waxes compromises lung health, so if you're a regular dabber, you should definitely be using dewaxed products most of the time. Winterized shatter also produces a smoother vapor because of the further removal of heavy waxes.

Winterization was actually one of the early methods for cleaning open-blasted BHO before extractors embraced vacuum drying as the industry standard for purging. That said, it should not be used as an alternative to a proper vacuum purge.

For chemical winterization, freshly extracted BHO with some solvent in it, (enough that it's still runny) is poured directly into 99.5% or purer ethanol and frozen by placing the containment vessel into a cooler full of chopped dry ice. In a few minutes the solution will freeze, exposing the plant wax to cold temperatures and causing it to sink to the bottom, where it can be skimmed out.

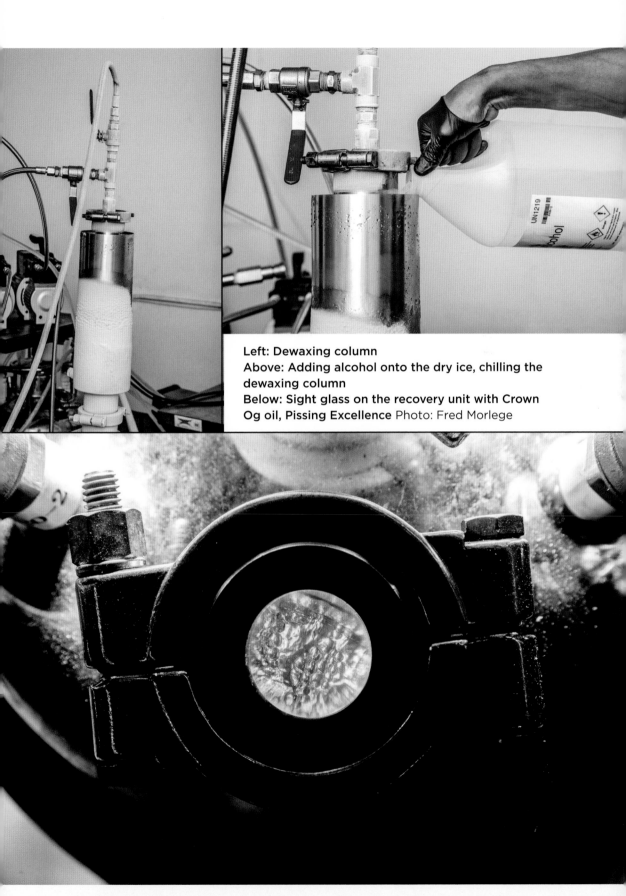

Left: Dewaxing column
Above: Adding alcohol onto the dry ice, chilling the dewaxing column
Below: Sight glass on the recovery unit with Crown Og oil, Pissing Excellence Photo: Fred Morlege

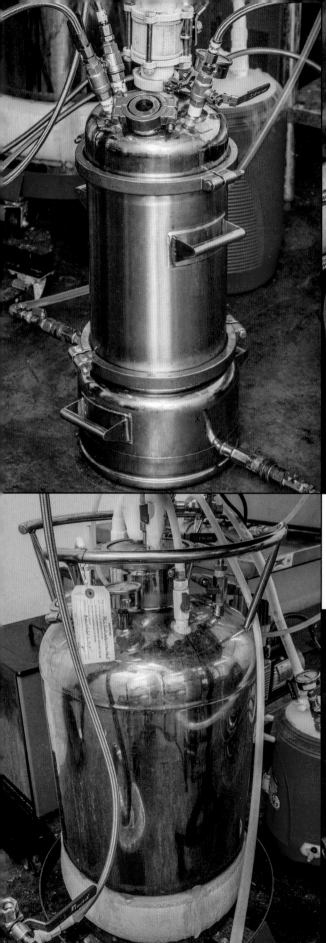

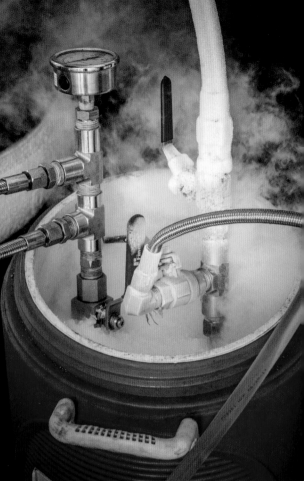

Top left: Recovery tank
Above: Condensing coil
Left: Butane solvent tank
Below: Bottom of a recovery tank after the butane has been recovered but before it has been purged.

Crown OG live resin, Pissing Excellence
Photos: Fred Morlege

Some closed-loop systems have recapture units that offer "in-line winterization," which is a special stage in the process where the raw solution sits in a steel drum surrounded by a layer of dry ice. The dry ice flash freezes the drum and the waxes in the off-gassing BHO collect on its sides.

Another simple method is to flash freeze your buds directly before extraction. This will allow for slightly longer passes (and larger yields) without compromising color or quality by slowing the release of lipids. We suggest at least one of these three methods be used; freezing your material, chemical winterization, or freezing your column. Most extractors do not do all three.

The product of an open-loop system can also be winterized using dry ice or a Buchner — a glass beaker funnel fitted with a super chilled 1.5-micron pumice stone. For dry ice, place slabs of ice underneath the Pyrex dish used to catch the raw solution during extraction. The cold from the dry ice will cause the waxes and lipids to sink to the bottom of the Pyrex and congeal on it. Dump the remaining dewaxed solution into a clean Pyrex dish.

For a Buchner, the raw solution is poured into the Buchner funnel, and the vacuum pump is used to pull the BHO through the cold stone matrix, which holds on to the waxes while the rest of the solution falls through into the Erlenmeyer flask.

SAFETY WARNING ON WINTERIZING

Sticking a mason jar full of liquid butane solution in the freezer isn't winterizing — it's bomb making. Thankfully, the addition of ethanol abates the explosion risk completely. However, it still presents a serious fire hazard because of ethanol's highly flammable nature. Make sure to avoid open flames around the area where you're winterizing — this includes pilot lights.

BHO STYLE BREAKDOWN

- Wax
- Honeycomb
- Budder/Badder
- Crumble
- Shatter
- Pull 'n' snap
- Sugar
- Live resin
- Terp crystals

PURGING

The initial result of BHO extraction is a solution of solvent and actual extract. Because of its physical properties, much of the butane will "boil off" at room temperature — this is technically the first purge — but additional purging is still required to remove residuals and achieve one of the many possible products.

One analogy is candy making: The ingredients and preparation for a lollipop are practically identical to those for a stick of taffy, the big difference being the temperature they are raised to — slightly cooler for taffy and a bit hotter for hard candy. BHO is similar; it always starts with a solution of extract and solvent, and the way the mixture is processed determines the final product. It's important to keep in mind that a proper purge can take several days and a lot of patience.

There are two ways to prepare butane for storage: freezing or squeezing. The freezing recapture entails cooling the gas enough to store it as a liquid, while squeezing involves using pressure to return butane to its liquid state for storage. Use the vacuum pump on the extractor to perform the second purge — reclaiming your solvent. Extraction machine makers often modify the collection chamber with a double wall to flow warm water (68°F [20°C] tops) around it to speed the recovery of the solvent.

Heat is the enemy of extraction. High temperature ruins shatter. Heat evaporates the terpenes that give great BHO its smell and flavors. Terpenes begin to evaporate at 68°F (20°C). Heat promotes hash decarboxylation, turning it into a dark oil suitable only for making edibles. Pay special attention to heat at all times.

After the initial purge, the material will no longer be a transparent liquid but a thick, goopy, runny toothpaste. Extractors remove the material drier or wetter, depending on their goals of making shatter, oil, or "crude oil" for distillates.

Dump the goop into a Pyrex dish, then scrape it onto a sheet of parchment paper. Fold the sheets into little trays with 2- to 3-inch walls. Preheat the oven to 94°F–98°F (34°C–37°C).

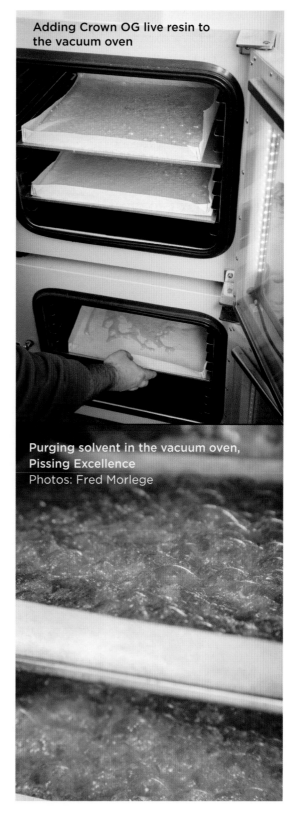

Adding Crown OG live resin to the vacuum oven

Purging solvent in the vacuum oven, Pissing Excellence
Photos: Fred Morlege

Now it's time to apply gentle heat under low pressure to finish purging and processing the batch. BHO is categorized by consistency, with shatter and "sugar" generally being the most prized. Next comes honeycomb, budder, wax, and oil.

The goal should be to produce the driest, lightest color BHO possible. Good-quality shatter is clear like yellow or amber glass and breaks at room temperature, whereas high-quality honeycomb (wax) is very pale, opaque, or translucent, dry and crumbly. Budder has a warm taffy quality to it, while oil is viscous and tacky. Sugar should have a sandy, granular consistency, a translucent clarity and a slightly wet look and feel.

A NOTE ON LIVE RESIN

Some methods for producing full-spectrum terpene extracts involve running the extractor at cold temperatures, allowing the processor to utilize fresh frozen material, still very high in aromatics and terpenoids. The result is a sappy rich sauce that smells like the starting product. Sauces command a very high per-gram price on the open market.

Live resin extractions and purging, which utilize fresh or fresh frozen plant material instead of cured, is covered in its own chapter. That chapter also covers "diamond mining" and other BHO methods, because most of them utilize live resin as their base.

Mendo Breath shatter , Pissing Excellence
Photo: Fred Morlege

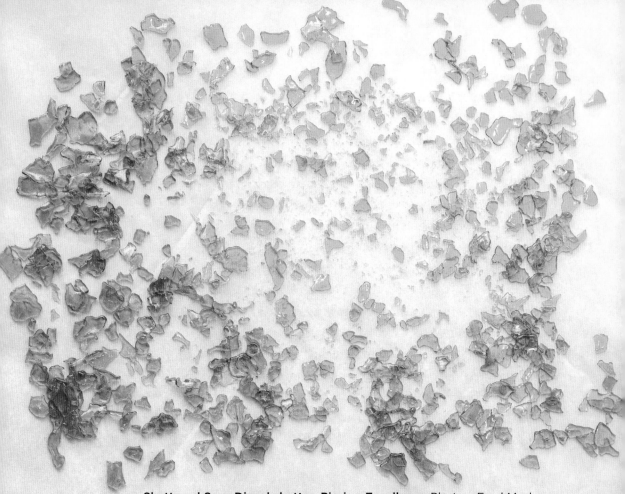

Shattered Sour Diesel shatter, Pissing Excellence Photos: Fred Morlege

VACUUM OVEN BASICS: SHATTER, WAX, BUDDER, AND DISTILLATE

Temperatures and vacuum settings can vary widely. Torr or mm Hg is a measure of pressure: the ratio of force to the area over which that force is distributed; mm Hg refers to milligrams of mercury, but a more common measure in America would be pounds per square inch, or psi. Pressure measurement converters are available online and -600 mm Hg (Torr) equals -11.6 psi.

SHATTER

The tastes of cannabis consumers are ever changing. One month the market demands crystal clarity; the next, consumers want terp crystals. There's no reliable way to predict which way the cannabis market will shift, so it's best to dial in an effective process and master it.

With that in mind, shatter is the most difficult consistency to achieve, but it's one that consistently enjoys steady demand; get this style right, and the demand will be a reliable safe haven from the always shifting tastes for other styles.

HOW TO MAKE SHATTER

As with all styles of BHO, start by placing the pre-purged resin on parchment paper and place it on a rack in a specialized vacuum oven set to 98°F with a minimum pressure setting of -600 mm Hg — use more pull if possible. Do not use a normal vacuum oven — butane will degrade typical vacuum pumps, so use one specialized to withstand exposure to liquid butane. The purge process will take from 24 to 36 hours and should be interrupted at least twice by "slab flipping," which will mechanically release more solvent through exposure of alternating surfaces to heat.

The residual butane in the solution is too low to present any fire hazard, but as the pressure drops and the temperature rises, the material will visibly "loaf up." This is normal. You can drop the "muffin" by opening the mantle. If the extractor hasn't pre-purged enough residual butane, the process must be stopped. You can get transparent clarity by pulling the vacuum harder, but it will reduce the operating life of your pump.

Another key aspect of the purge process is lowering the viscosity of the slab to allow more solvent to escape. The key to getting this right is to monitor the bubbles; keep an eye out for big, thin bubbles that pop themselves without assistance. If the bubbles are thick and don't pop, the viscosity hasn't been reduced enough and the temperature setting should be boosted. Or, if there is no expansion or off-gassing the heat may be set too high — the entire process is a delicate balancing act.

Even within the classification of "shatter" there are several subsets of texture, ranging from flexible saps to malleable and brittle "snap 'n' pull" shatters. For strains that yield a sappy consistency, the heat setting could be as low as 68°F, but for the snap 'n' pull, it will measure between 85°F and 100°F. Classic shatter — the hard golden resin with solid stability and crystal clarity — will heat to 95°F to 115°F. Some strains will require up to 120°F, but over 112°F will cause most strains to "budder."

WAX AND BUDDERING

Leaving shatter in the vac oven at 110°F–120°F for several hours results in a honeycomb-like wafer. More butane is removed when the temperature is raised and the pressure lowered, but this also removes more terpenes.

But if shatter turns from clear to opaque, a process called nucleation (or "buddering") has occurred. The process is more or less a one-way street: Once a shatter "budders up," it must go through another process to get it back to true shatter.

Shatter turns to budder when heated too long or exposed to contaminants like residual water. Even the finest shatter turns to budder eventually during storage: "Buddered" extracts are the result of a process called nucleation. An example of this process can be seen in an old milk chocolate bar: the surface takes on a powdery white patina from the separation of milk fats and

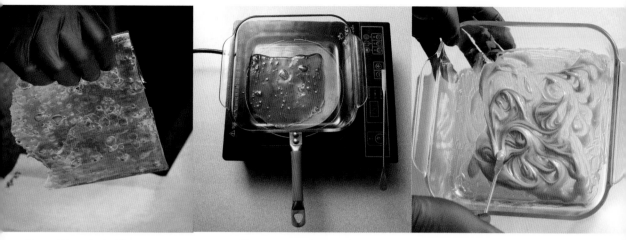

Sour Diesel shatter

Shatter on a pyrex hot plate melting down

Whipped into butter

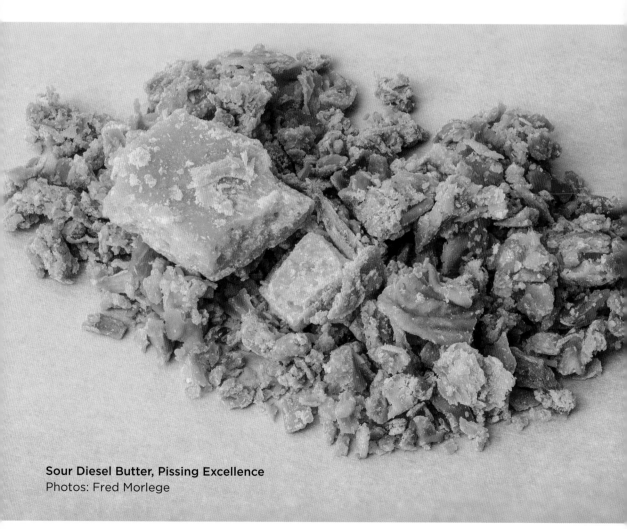

Sour Diesel Butter, Pissing Excellence
Photos: Fred Morlege

Honeycomb close up from Oakland Extracts

Crumble cookies created with Cookie Tech by Oakland Extracts creates easy to handle crumble that resembles vanilla wafers.

sugar, and the consistency is chalky and crumbly. In shatter, heavier fats and lipids precipitate out of the solution. Buddering often starts in one corner of the resin patty and spreads across the entire piece.

Today's market is fickle. One day clarity and stability are the most desirable trait; the next, it might be terpene concentration. Nucleated shatter often has a much "louder" terpene profile than the shatter it started as, so don't worry too much if nucleation strikes a shatter slab. As long as the BHO has been extracted and purged properly, retaining the flavor profile and cannabinoid content while removing residual hydrocarbons, the other physical characteristics are a matter of taste.

DISTILLATE

Distillate is enjoying an increase in popularity because of its potency — upward of 90% cannabinoid concentration — and because it's flavorless, though the addition of food-grade or re-claimed cannabis terpenes allows for customization. The process is simple enough — winter-ized oil is poured into a short-path distillation system, which allows for "fractional distillation." For more in-depth information on short path and fractional distillation, see the "Distillate" chapter.

DECARBOXYLATION OF BHO

Because it is an extraction of THCa, BHO is not psychoactive in its raw form. It is completely harmless in this form if it is accidentally ingested by a pet, a child, or an unaware adult. However, THCa offers many medical benefits to people who want relief without euphoria.

If the BHO is to be used in edibles, it must first be decarboxylated—a process through which THCa and/or CBDa turns into THC and CBD. This starts happening at 222°F (106°C).

Thankfully, it's quite easy to decarboxylate purged BHO — just double boil it in a water bath set to above 222°F (106°C). The BHO will start producing CO_2 bubbles when it exceeds the target temperature, at which point it must be stirred. When the bubbles taper off, the BHO is decarboxylated.

But be careful: The same heat that turns THCa into THC also turns THC into cannabinol (CBN), which produces a more sedative effect than THC. When THCa is 70% decarboxylated into THC, the rate of THC-to-CBN production eclipses the rate of decarboxylation from THCa to THC. That is, when the bubble formation tapers off, the oil has reached the maximum level of THC, and further heat will only increase CBN and make it more sedative.

Of course, BHO destined to be dabbed or vaped doesn't require decarboxylation — the heat used during consumption will take care of that process.

Extraction Tek Solutions

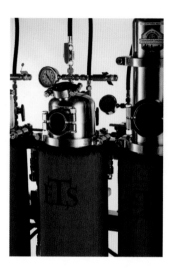

"Necessity is the mother of invention" comes to mind if you delve into the history of ExtractionTek Solutions (ETS). When founder Matthew Ellis started experimenting with closed-loop extraction systems for butane, he wasn't necessarily looking for a more efficient means of producing cannabis extracts. His primary concern was to address a widespread hazard in the industry – open air hydrocarbon extraction, or "open blasting."

By the time Ellis started designing a closed-loop butane extraction system, he had many years of experience with other types of extraction systems. In 2008, he became fascinated with the field, and took it upon himself to learn everything he could on the subject. Soon after, he co-founded Organa Labs, Colorado's first licensed manufacturer of infused products to develop cannabis products, using an Eden Labs CO_2 extraction system.

Over the course of his career, he has worked with hundreds of active extraction operations, and through these partnerships and shared development, he has been able to build the client focused solutions and training methods that the industry demands.

So when Ellis saw an opportunity to design a safer, more reliable method of hydrocarbon extraction, he decided to team up with Marcus Fauth to build the first professional-grade, ETL listed closed loop hydrocarbon extraction system. The ETS 1300™ was the company's flagship product, and ExtractionTek Solutions was launched in 2011.

The company's core mission was to develop and manufacture the industry's leading hydrocarbon extraction systems, which are as safe as they are reliable. As of July 2016, ETS was awarded United States Design Patents for all three models in its production line. All three ETS machines enjoy the smallest machine footprint in their capacity categories -- no other machine in the industry can process more material within a 5'x3' footprint.

Product consistency is key to the long-term success of any extraction operation, and ETS machines offer their operators flexibility in process without sacrificing consistency or safety requirements. Most important, all of the company's equipment meets or exceeds regulatory requirements for all legal regulated cannabis markets. ExtractionTek also services and supports all of its extraction equipment, and offers a full suite of training services to ensure safety and proper operation. If companies that want to extend their capacity, the company's Modular Extraction Platform can be adjusted and scaled to meet future production demands.

ExtractionTek Solutions manufacturers all of its machines using only high-quality U.S. manufactured steel and components, and all of it units and accessories are peer reviewed. From the very beginning, ETS has held itself to a high standard, and that ethic remains a steady force in its current company culture.

"It all comes down to an incredible amount of effort and passion pursued by a small group of friends and family to make a product we knew the world needed," says Ellise. "We push that boulder together with purpose and discipline and hold ourselves and our company to a higher standard than our competitors. Our clients have grown to be an important piece of our company's culture, and we wear that honor proudly and guard that trust carefully."

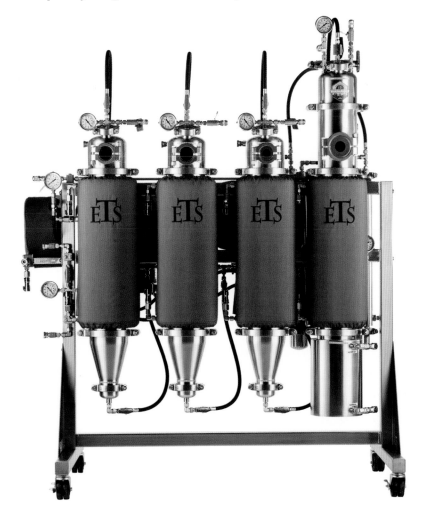

A pancake made with live resin extraction by Ascent Extracts. DEA licensed test results of Ascent's live resin showed a 97.21% total cannabinoid content purity with over 35 different terpenes and cannabinoids.

CHAPTER 4

BHO 201: Live Resin

It's impossible to cover *every* cannabis extraction method being used, in small part because so many different techniques are still in the process of being developed. All the methods covered in this book correlate with widely used industrial processes rooted in basic organic chemistry, but their application to cannabis is relatively new.

There are plenty of extractors who rely solely on the methods covered in the previous chapter — basic hydrocarbon extraction using cured material — and there's no shortage of consumers who are perfectly satisfied with standard hydrocarbon products made using cured cannabis. However, as the focus of connoisseur consumers has shifted heavily toward terpene profiles, extractors have been exploring ways to maximize the terpene levels of their products. One of the primary methods for achieving this is the use of "live" material — buds that have just been harvested or which were flash frozen immediately after harvest — instead of cured buds that have been processed for smoking. This process (and the other techniques covered in this section) requires a bit more precision, but when performed properly the result will be more flavorful and sometimes more aesthetically striking.

As we delve into some of the more advanced methods of producing solvent-extracted cannabis concentrates, it's important to keep in mind that there are no "secret techniques" when it comes to extraction — this is all basic organic chemistry. Some extractors have perfected their own semi-proprietary procedure for harnessing that chemistry, but using the information in this section, you can produce most of the currently popular expressions of BHO, including "terp sauce" and "diamonds" of THCa.

LIVE RESIN

Butane extraction with properly cured source material produces cured resin, a product with an extremely potent flavor profile. But as the taste of cannabis consumers has developed to demand even stronger terpene expressions, many extractors are turning to live or fresh frozen material to produce live resin, which not only has a "louder" terpene profile but also lends itself more readily to creating highly desirable sugars and other crystallized concentrates.

Like cured resin, live resin can take a variety of physical forms. The elevated terpene content is associated with buddering and crystallization, but that doesn't mean it's impossible to make excellent, stable shatter using live material. All shatter will nucleate eventually over time; there's no way to prevent it. Processes such as dewaxing and winterizing provide additional stability and forestall the onset of nucleation. However, these techniques also reduce terpene concentration, which is why the prevailing practice is to produce sugars and terp sauces using live resin.

There are methods for refining and repairing subpar BHO (see short-path distillation), but harnessing the full potential of solvent extraction means sourcing flavorful, potent cannabis, and to that end fresher is always better. This is also true of cured material: trimmed and cured bud will never be as fresh as frozen live bud, because it's essential to preserve the terpene profile.

There is no cured substitute for a dab of fresh, well-crafted live resin. The drying and curing process, though crucial to the preparation of smokable bud, is often destructive when it comes to terpenes. Most cannabis smokers have experienced the disappointment of finding some forgotten bud, only to discover that the once robust flavor profile has been replaced with a harsh, unsatisfying smoke. That doesn't mean there aren't well-cured buds that retain their terpene profiles, and there are plenty of cured resins that fully express that flavor.

The fresher the material the better, even with cured bud, but it doesn't get any fresher than just harvested, which is precisely why extractors started experimenting with live and fresh frozen material in the first place. Any successful extraction effort means getting the freshest material possible, but live resin demands the retention and preservation of precious terpenes. Even if the material can't be processed immediately, proper freezing will generally provide a much more flavorful product than cured material.

Freezing the starting material is always beneficial, even when using cured buds or trim, because freezing isolates the water soluble elements that can reduce butane's efficiency as a solvent.

It is technically possible to utilize fresh trim for this process, but every time the plant is cut, it creates more opportunities for chlorophyll to leach into the resin during extraction. This is the reason early attempts at live resin often resulted in products with greenish colors. If the material is mostly untrimmed and properly frozen, chlorophyll and other water soluble elements are locked out of the extraction process, creating a cleaner, more flavorful product. Avoid breaking up the buds — trim them individually at the stem.

The basics of freezing the material are simple: Chop it down, bag it up, vacuum seal it, and place the bags on dry ice. This should also be done with cured material for the same basic reasons; we're trying to prevent the evaporation of terpenes.

Because freshness is key when extracting live resin, avoid much trimming — even wet trimming, which in addition to delaying freezing releases chlorophyll through the cuts. When using outside material, make sure the source knows what's needed in terms of freshness and freezing. It does make sense to remove large fan leaves, but keep most of the guard leaves. Remove yellow or brown leaves and anything that's been cut or bitten by insects, then immediately freeze. Large quantities can take up to 36 hours in a freezer set at -10°F or below.

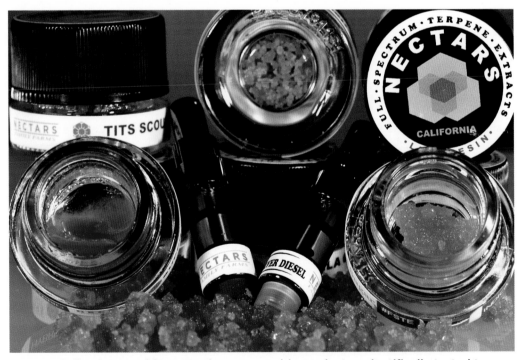

Nectars Collective provides connoisseur cannabis products, scientifically tested to ensure the highest standards of purity. Their Terp Juice sets the bar high, with lab tested results showing levels of terpenes ranging from 18 - 37%.

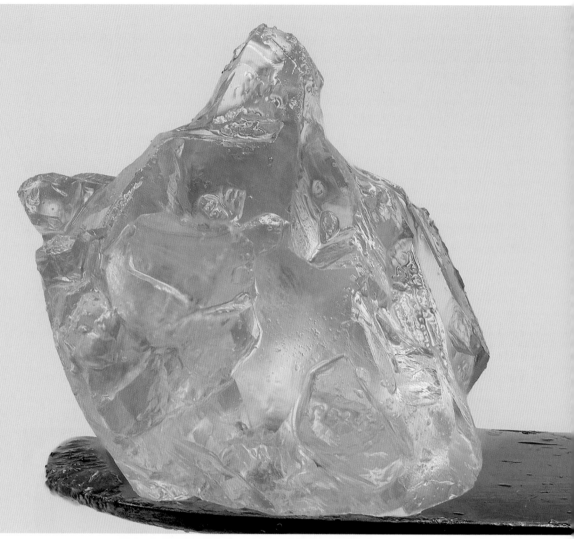

A single diamond of crystallized THC-A from a batch of Albert Walker Live Resin, Marquise Diamond Series by First Class Concentrates

LIVE RESIN BASICS

Here are some basic tips to keep in mind when attempting live resin extraction:

- **Freshness is everything** — Freshness is fundamentally what distinguishes live resin from cured resin, so it's impossible to overstate the importance. The starting material needs to be the freshest, highest quality possible.
- **Be speedy** — The less time spent cleaning up the plant, the less delay between chopping it down and freezing it., This process should be completed in an hour or less to avoid loss of terpenes.
- **Buds are best** — Using trim is not advisable when making live resin.
- **Cold is the key** — solvent extraction requires keeping the process cold and this is doubly true when extracting live resin. Maintaining the true terpene profile of

the source material leaves little margin for error, so controlling the temperature of the process and keeping it within target zones for terpene preservation is absolutely crucial. Ideally, live resin extraction is cold all the way through.

FREEZING LIVE MATERIAL

There are multiple methods for freezing fresh buds, but by far the simplest is to bag them and put the bags in a deep freezer at 10°F or colder. Some other methods call for flash freezing the buds, but since you're starting from live material, a gradual freeze will effectively preserve the terpenes, making faster methods unnecessary. Whatever method you use, the best practice is to extract the material within 36 hours of freezing — ideally, you'll extract it immediately after it freezes.

Because ethanol and ice are used throughout much of the extraction process, many closed-loop extractors use them to create a cooling bath for flash freezing their starting material in a jacketed closed loop collection pot. Here's what you'll need:

MAKING A DRY ICE COOLING BATH

MATERIALS

- Metal or rubber container — do not use glass or plastic
- Gloves and eye protection — ethanol can splash and burn skin, dry ice must be handled with gloves
- Ethanol — the higher the concentration, the colder the bath: 70% is fine, but 100% will freeze the material the fastest
- Dry ice

Preparing the bath

1. Carefully break the dry ice into manageable chunks and place them in the container
2. Pour ethanol over the dry ice, slowly to avoid splashing, until the ice is covered
3. Add more ice or ethanol as needed when boiling activity slows

Now that the dry ice bath is ready, it's time to freeze the buds. Don't just drop them into the bath. Seal them inside vacuum bags, making sure to arrange the material to maximize the surface area for even freezing.

1. Fill vacuum bags with buds — arrange for maximum surface area
2. Purge humidity from bags with dry ice
3. Vacuum seal bags
4. Dip bag into cooling bath until frozen — the freezing time will depend on the amount of material being frozen

COOLING BUTANE

Regardless of the freezing method used, the butane will also need to be cooled. If it isn't, the frozen buds will just thaw out in the relatively warm butane, releasing lipids and undesirable chlorophyll.

Make a dry ice cooling bath and submerge a condensing coil in it. This should cool the butane down substantially, from -20°C to -50°C, depending on the concentration of the ethanol, the size of the bath, and the quantity of ice used. When the butane reaches the packed column, it will be cold enough to prevent thawing and preserve the terpenes.

Some extractors also freeze the column, which can be done separately or at the same time as the buds. If the bud is frozen already, utilize another ice bath, a cryogenic pump, or some other method to cool the tube and ensure that the buds do not thaw during extraction. The benefit to freezing the bud separately is the ability to process a larger quantity while storing the unused frozen bud during processing.

PURGING LIVE RESIN

Removing or "purging" residual solvent is a crucial step to BHO extraction, and live resin is no exception — all BHO must be processed to remove the extraction solvent still trapped inside.

Terpene concentration is central to the value of all concentrates, and terpenes are natural solvents, so the purge process is always a delicate dance between reaching safe levels of residual solvent without eliminating or diminishing the terpene concentration. Because terpenes are central to the appeal of live resin, this balancing act can be difficult.

The process of purging live resin isn't dramatically different from purging cured resin, except that you won't be flipping it if your end goal is a sugar consistency. One common approach is to heat the extract up to its target temperature before pulling gas into the vacuum oven. It also makes sense to purge at lower temperatures, with the understanding that this will increase the length of your purge process, sometimes by days. Ultimately, you'll need to dial in each strain to your system through a test batch and a trip to your local testing lab.

The key is to watch the bubbles in your purging resin through the vacuum oven view window. When the large bubbles subside and are replaced by smaller ones, you're finished. Just keep track of the time so you can adjust your approach if your test results come back with a high butane ratio.

And remember, don't go through all the effort of securing fresh material, freezing it, and keeping your extraction process quick and cold just to burn up your terps on the purge; keep the heat as low as possible — well under 110°F.

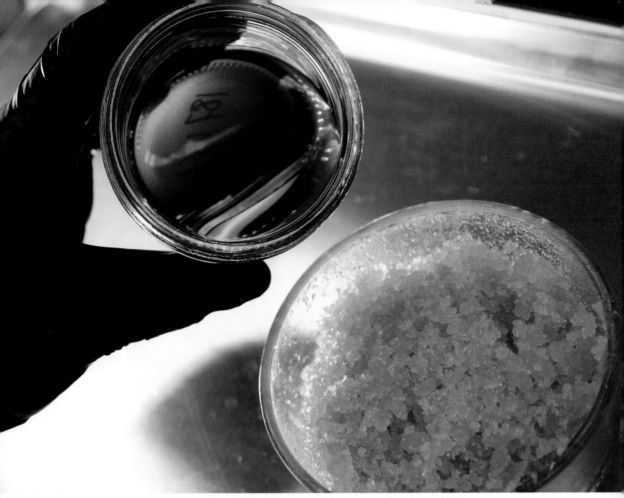

Live Nectar™ consists of terpene-rich sauce covering crystals of raw THCa.
Harmony Extracts

"DIAMOND MINING" OR "JAR TECH"

First and foremost — and stop us if you've heard this one before — this is all basic organic chemistry, in this case, a process called "recrystallization." There are several other names, two primary ones being Diamond Mining and Jar Tech, which refer to the end product and a technique for achieving it, respectively.

Diamond Mining is all about encouraging separation of cannabinoids from terpenes. It isn't as precise as fractional distillation, but the end product can be incredibly flavorful and potent, and many dabbers who prefer live resin also prefer the crystallization of "terp sauce."

Shatter made from live resin has a higher terpene concentration than cured resin, which tends to be more susceptible to nucleation, creating terp sugar or budder after it has been packaged. This was once seen as a liability, as it undermines the stability that consumers look for in a good shatter. Now that many cannabis consumers prefer the sugar consistency, extractors precrystallize their BHO.

The biggest appeal of live resin is the elevated terpene content that leads to the physical separation associated with sauces and sugars. The only problem is that once the product sep-

Molten sauce flows over geodes of THCa, reeking of Harmony's garden. Harmony Extracts

arates, the increased terpene concentration is only temporary. The sugar consistency is the result of solid cannabinoids separating from the liquid terpenes, lending a more robust aroma but resulting in rapid terpene loss through evaporation.

A WORD ON RECRYSTALLIZATION

This book primarily focuses on recrystallization methods for hydrocarbon extracts because the majority of commercially available recrystallized products are made using hydrocarbons. However, it is technically possible to recrystallize any cannabis concentrate that hasn't been decarboxylated; as long as there are cannabinoid acids present, they can be used to create crystalline structures. However, all the well-established methods of recrystallization require the use of solvent of some kind.

There are a variety of methods for producing a crystalline cannabis concentrate, including fractional distillation, but one of the simplest and most time-consuming involves little more than time and terpenes.

Diamond Mining can be done with cured resin, but live resin more readily lends itself to the process. As with all extraction, starting material is the key to everything that follows, and there are no short cuts or workarounds when it comes to this step — get the loudest, most potent cannabis available. Each strain has idiosyncratic qualities when it comes to resin stability, crystallization potential, and so on, and most of extraction is science, but this is one of those areas where it becomes something of an art form. Selecting the strain that best suits the desired end product is all about trial and error.

The process starts the same way all BHO products do — with butane extraction. Once you've extracted the unpurged live resin it's time to do a light, no-vac purge at roughly 90°F — no higher than 100°F. This will off-gas most, but not all, of the residual solvent. The resin is now placed into containers where it is left to separate for two to three weeks. During that time cannabinoid crystals start to form on the bottom of the container as the solids separate from the terpenes, forming a semiviscous liquid layer on top. When you're satisfied with the stacking of the crystals, it's time for the final purge.

If possible, separate the liquid layer from the crystals and purge them separately. The terpene layer will be more or less liquid, making it fairly easy to pour off. This allows for a slightly longer purge on the crystals, roughly 72 hours, versus 60 or so for the terp sauce. If for some reason your layers are difficult to separate, the entire batch can be purged together, but it should still be purged for less time than a shatter; shatter is generally purged for at least 100 hours, but with Diamond Mining, the resin has already been partially purged and has also been off-gassing in the container for weeks.

Once the purge is complete, the liquid and solid products are recombined and packaged, preferably in a UV-proof container to slow the loss of terpenes. The natural separation of cannabinoids and terpenes employed in this process are pronounced but not total. That means the terpene-rich semi-fluid portion will still contain anywhere from 30% to 50% cannabinoids.

"DIAMOND MINING" RECRYSTALLIZATION PROCESS BREAKDOWN

1. Extract some BHO from some quality material. Dried, cured buds work fine, but live resin is the best starting material.
2. When the BHO is still highly viscous, pour it into a mason jar. Place a lid on the jar.
3. Place the jar somewhere where it stays above room temperature, taking specific note of the formation of the crystalization. Slightly lower or higher temperatures can affect the length of the process or the overall size and clarity of the formations.

> Warning: It is highly likely the jar will need to be burped if heated above room temperature. The more heat you use in this step the faster the solvent converts to a gaseous form. You are are intentionally heating the material SLOWLY in an effort to mine as large and as clear a crystalline formation as you can. Adding more heat means more internal temperature in your jar. If your jar fails to hold the pressure it can shatter sending broken glass flying everywhere. Jars should be placed in a receptacle to minimize danger to the extractor. Always wear proper protective equipment.

4. You may need to vent pressure from your jar so that opening it when you check on it is just fine.
5. As time passes in this soupy pressurized state, THCa crystals begin to form and fall out of suspension to the bottom of the jar. The volatile terpenes rise to form a viscous layer on top of the mix in the jar.
6. When you're happy with the crystal formation, you can pour off the terps to separate the crystals.
7. Terpenes can be stabilized by purging, re-added to the crystals for flavor or made into their own dabbable product.
8. To further refine the THCa you can wash it in another hydrocarbon such as pentane to try to remove the remaining residual solvents.
9. Dab it.

OTHER LIVE RESIN CONSIDERATIONS

Nucleation may start before the packaging stage. In that case, encourage and speed up the process. This can be achieved with a double water bath and a little physical agitation if you notice buddering. If it's already showing crystallization, you can pop it in a container and try a modified Diamond Mining approach.

Live resin can provide a more flavorful product, but with a few exceptions the process is no different from extracting cured resin. Since live resin lends itself more readily to crystallization, it's a perfect choice if you're looking to focus on sugars and terp sauces instead of shatters.

Finally, remember that there are two basic approaches to extraction. The original approach, which inspired the name of this book's predecessor *Trash to Stash*, is all about taking trim and other less desirable parts of the cannabis plant (or less successful crops) and turning them into something that still provides high potency. The newer approach is about condensing and highlighting desirable elements in quality material — live resin falls squarely in this category. There's no wrong way to approach the processing of cannabis, as long as you have a clear picture of where you're trying to go. For those seeking a way to process large quantities of larf, live resin is a dead end. For those focusing almost exclusively on terpene profiles, it's a golden ticket.

Almost 400 grams of Harmony Mars OG Live Nectar™. Harmony Extracts

Across International

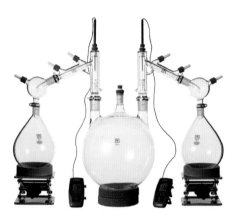

One of the critical steps in the manufacturing process for cannabis extracts is purging the solvents that are used in the (initial) extraction process.. When done correctly, this vacuum purging results in a safe, clean and pure product, among the most coveted of which are terpene-rich, tasty BHO products.

Across International (Ai) was founded as a company that sold laboratory equipment to R&D facilities, universities, government agencies, and other businesses. So when they discovered that their vacuum and distillation equipment was being used by cannabis extractors, it came as something of a pleasant surprise.

"Since then, we have been driven to develop technology to further medical cannabis research and provide dispensaries with equipment that substantially improves the quality of their end products," says Maxwell Dubin. "We embrace the cannabis industry and truly enjoy working with so many talented professionals."

Across International manufactures everything that's needed for extraction-related processes, including winterization, filtration, simple and fractional distillation, homogenization, and solvent purging. By using their vacuum ovens, pumps, rotary evaporators and distillation kits, producers can effectively capture and re-condense terpenes, purify oils, and quickly freeze plant and liquid materials. Vacuum ovens, for instance, are used to put oil under an atmospheric pressure in an airtight chamber, which lowers the boiling point of each of the compounds, most importantly the residual solvents, within the BHO (and other solvent extractions, or water from CO_2 and rosin extractions). This process allows certain compounds to be cold boiled away without damaging others.

For short path distillation, a boiling flask is heated in a mantle under vacuum pressure. The distillate then travels a short distance before recondensing, which ensures that the least amount of compound is lost on the sides of the apparatus. This process is used for batch purification, which is achieved with multiple passes at different temperatures.

Headquartered and founded in Livingston, New Jersey, Across International brings more than 25 years of industrial equipment manufacturing experience to the cannabis market. The company attended its first Cannabis Cup was in 2014, and has won numerous awards over the years for its equipment, including the High Times S.T.A.S.H. (Significant Technological Achievements in Secretive Horticulture), Gear of the Year in 2013, 2014, and 2015, and the ExpoGrow Best Paraphernalia Product in 2015.

Across International strives for the highest quality in its manufacturing and is in the process of completing UL / CSA certification for all of its instruments. They use PTFE food-grade seals on their distillation glassware and offer both Silicone and Viton for their vacuum ovens.. All of their products have multiple size options, so operators can start small and scale up to mass production over time. Due to the high demand for their products, Across International now has more than 200 distributors worldwide. Quality control, replacement parts, warranty and repair services, and customer support is all provided in the USA.

Outside of cannabis industry, Across International works with university and government agencies, and has an impressive B2B customer base that includes NASA, 3M, Tesla, and Lockheed Martin.

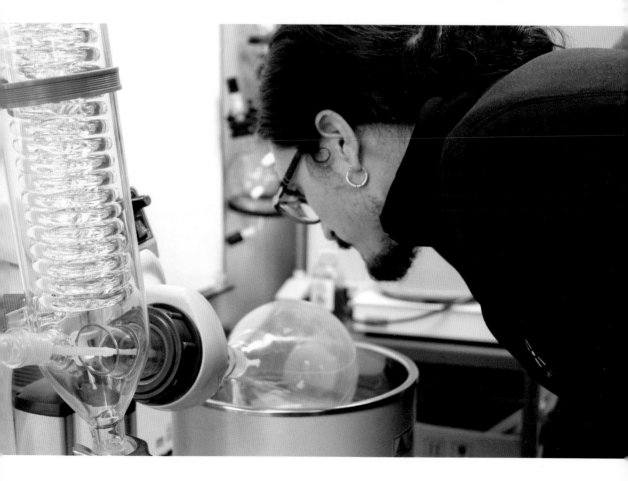

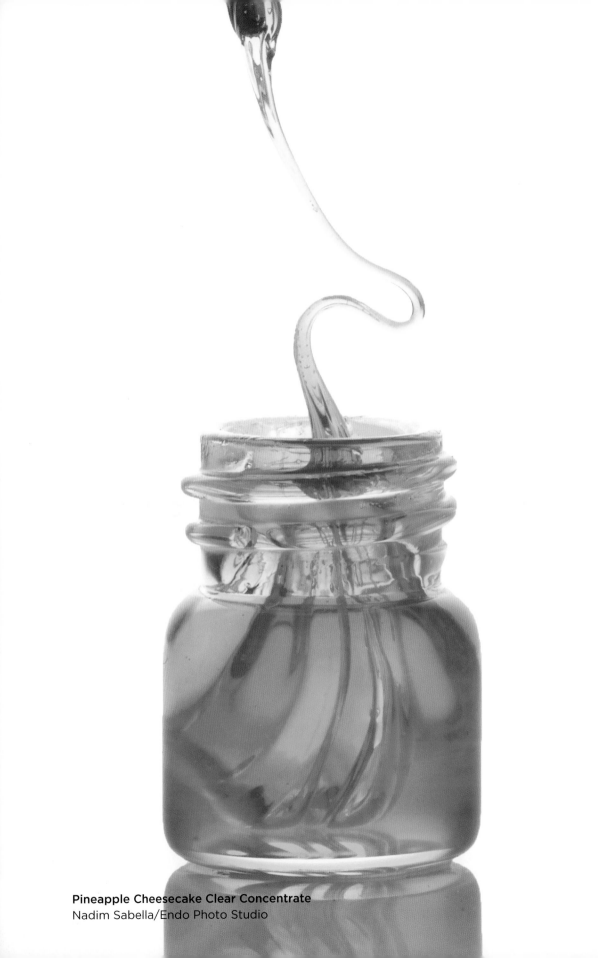

Pineapple Cheesecake Clear Concentrate
Nadim Sabella/Endo Photo Studio

Fractional and Short-Path Distillation

The Cutting Edge of Concentration Technology

One of this book's primary goals is demystifying processes that, in the end, amount to nothing more than basic organic chemistry. Of all the facets of cannabis extraction, none is quite so opaque to the general public as fractional distillation, a cornerstone of industrial extraction that is perceived by the cannabis world as prohibitively cutting edge — an arcane art practiced exclusively by alchemical sorcerers.

In reality, fractional distillation is merely a refinement of the ancient practice of simple distillation—a practice only slightly more complicated than boiling water. But before we dive into the simple science of distillation, let's talk about why it's being adopted by extractors and what kinds of products can be created using the end product.

DISTILLED CANNABIS PRODUCTS

Cannabis concentrates produced using most methods in this book will already have relatively high cannabinoid levels. Anything extracted using hydrocarbon solvents should test no lower than 60% THC, with more potent runs regularly reaching concentrations as high as 80% THC. So why refine them even further?

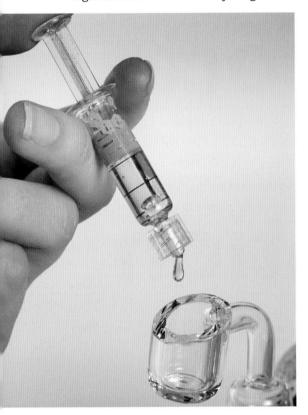

Sold in a convenient "dablicator," Next Level Labs produces a cannabis oil with a complex blend of terpenes added to precise cannabis ratios using fractional distillation techniques.

There are two primary reasons: the first is a desire for a superpotent (upward of 90% THC) product that is already "activated" and can be consumed orally, applied topically, or inhaled through vaping, dabbing, or even smoking. As with any of the methods in this book, as long as you responsibly source your material and maintain safe, clean laboratory conditions, the end product should be as safe to consume as any other cannabis concentrate.

The second reason for choosing distillation is a need to "repair" an undesirable run of cheap extract, which is often called "crude" oil when it's deliberately produced for use in distillation. Crude extract isn't particularly tasty or attractive; it's generally dark brown or black and has a sap-py, viscous consistency that makes it hard to work with at room temperature, but it still contains relatively high concentrations of THC (roughly 60%–80%) and can be used as the starting material for the distillation process. This crude extract can be purchased at basement prices too, so if you perfect the distillation process and find a market for the end product, it's not expensive to establish a supply chain.

Any extraction method with an eye toward terpene retention is based on a balancing act, meaning that there's always the possibility that something could upset that balance and compromise the end product. Sometimes that means a less flavorful or attractive product that can

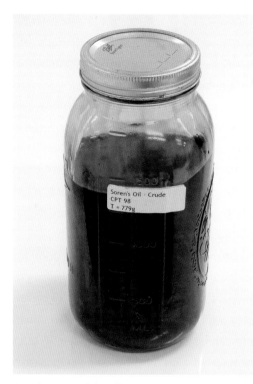

Crude cannabis oil, 779 grams before distilling at Next Level Labs. Photo: Ed Rosenthal

still be consumed or sold; taste is subjective, and not all consumers are as focused on flavor or appearances, so darker product with a less-pronounced terpene profile can still find a home somewhere without further processing.

Other times the end product of a failed extraction run is so undesirable that it simply can't be used as is — but all is not lost! This "crude" cannabis oil can still be salvaged through distillation, and while lost terpenes can't be resurrected, botched concentrates still contain intact cannabinoids that can be isolated through distillation. In fact, because of its hyperselective properties, short-path fractional distillation also removes pesticide and other residual contaminants, making it an ideal option for salvaging a tainted run.

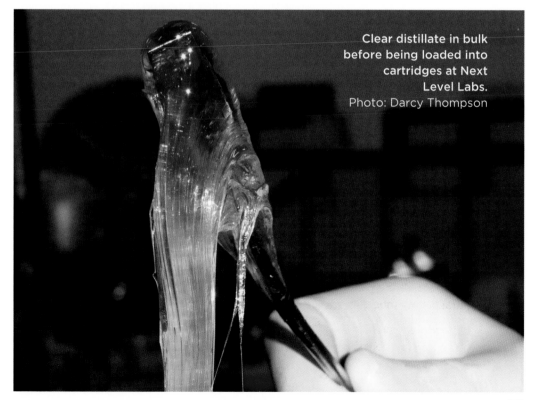

Clear distillate in bulk before being loaded into cartridges at Next Level Labs.
Photo: Darcy Thompson

DISTILLATE

One of the most visible expressions of this process is "clear" distillate, a viscous oil that's generally pale yellow or colorless, with a near-transparent clarity that lends the product its name. Its striking aesthetics are certainly an improvement on the dark sludge that often goes into producing it, but what's more remarkable than the appearance of distillate is its pronounced potency — often nearing 98% cannabinoid concentration. Additionally, because the process of distillation involves high enough heat to trigger decarboxylation, cannabis distillate is an "active" product that can be consumed orally or sublingually. However, it's particularly prized by dabbers focused on maximizing cannabinoid consumption. Where a dab of typical BHO or CO_2 shatter might contain 70–80% potency, distillate regularly hits 91% and higher, making it a powerful delivery system for instant cannabinoid impacts.

Clear distillate with terpenes re-added has also proved an immensely popular option for pre-filling vaporizer cartridges. The high potency makes it an ideal choice for those seeking to discretely and quickly consume concentrate on the go, and the same process used to isolate the distillate can also be used to extract the terpenes, which can be re-added to the product. Many producers use food-grade terpenes to mimic cannabis flavor profiles or simply offer candy and fruit flavoring for their carts. Not everyone is sold on inhaling artificial flavoring, but for many consumers the addition of familiar flavors enhances the pleasure of vaporizing concentrates.

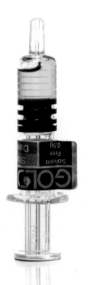

Gold Drop's dablicator contains a translucent, refined, solvent-free distillate oil that is odorless and flavorless and can be dabbed, added to a joint, blunt, or bowl.

Whether you're looking to medicate edibles, fill cartridges, or package distillate for dabbing, it's important to keep in mind these three key points about the process of distilling concentrates:

- The process destroys terpenes, so if you want to preserve them, it must be done before THC distillation.
- The process produces a decarboxylated "active" product.
- Performed properly, the process removes all pesticide and other residual impurities.

In addition to the more common viscous distillate, there are also crystalline cannabinoid solids — most notably THCa and CBDa that are available commerically. They range in concentration of 91% cannabinoid up to about 97% purity. Crystalline THCa has the appearance of a coarse, yellow powder. As the concentration climbs closer to 99.9%, the crystalline structure of the solids is visible without magnification; the resulting crystals resemble large chunks of rock salt.

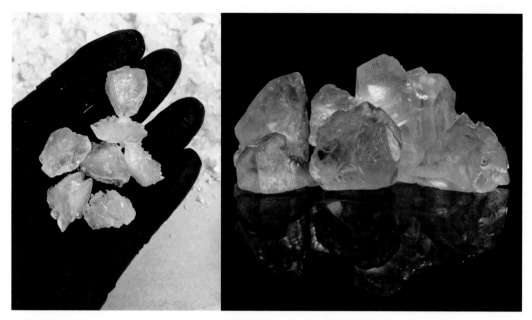

Left: THCa Crystalline extracted by Guild Extracts is 99%-100% THCa , making it one of the purest forms you can get. THCa converts to THC when vaped and creates a clear and highly cerebral effect but remains nonpsychoactive when ingested.
Right: THCa isolate produced at Harmony Extracts.

CRYSTALLIZATION

As with distillation, the process of crystallization/recrystallization is often seen as quasi-magical. It's really just the final step in isolating an organic compound. These isolates are powerful individually but do not contain their companion cannabinoids. That can be very desirable, as in the case of CBD users seeking its health benefits without a high. There is something exquisitely beautiful about these amazing compounds both in appearance and in potency.

These crystalline solid products have proved popular, albeit less so than the more accessible (and slightly easier to produce) clear distillates. There is an increased cost associated with the production of such refined concentrates, and that cost translates to higher retail prices that don't always appeal to consumers. Additionally, hyper-refined concentrates have a weakness hidden in their strength; the absence of terpenes to "inform" the effects of the cannabinoids means the detectable impacts of consumption are often less pronounced than expected. This has to do with the entourage effect and the way cannabis compounds work in concert to produce impacts in the human body. So in order to get the full benefit of these distilled products, the addition of terpenes has proved central for many consumers.

This has led extractors to offer combinations of crystalline cannabinoids and extracted terpenes, packaged together for easy consumption. While these types of products can be produced using distillation by extracting viscous, high-terpene concentrate and crystalline cannabinoid solids separately and combining them, the most desirable features of the end product can be achieved through less complex means, namely recrystallization, which is covered in the "Live Resin" chapter.

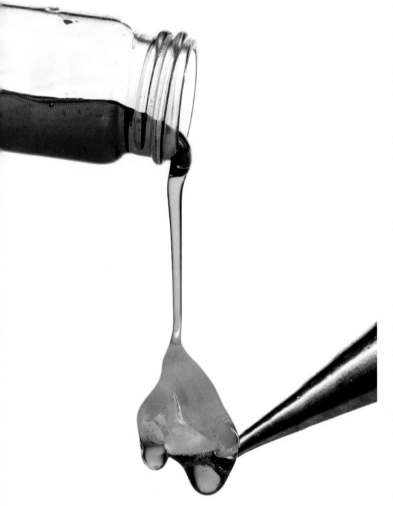

Distillation offers immense benefits to cannabis extractors, as a restorative/reparative process for subpar extracts or as a planned end game for raw material. The journey of discovery around cannabis extraction will never end, but we've reached the physical ceiling where potency is concerned: You can't get any purer than 100%, and we've pretty much achieved that using distillation. However, as with all other extraction methods, there's a sprawling sea of variables between the theoretical science and the practical application. Navigating that sea is where the artistry of extraction comes into play.

Before we dive into the physical particulars of fractional distillation as it applies to cannabis concentrates, let's acquaint ourselves with the basic chemistry behind simple distillation.

Adding terpenes to crystaline means that the dab will give you the taste experience of the whole flower. Harmony Extracts Nectar is made by isolating THCa, isolating the terpenes, then adding the terpenes back in liquid form.

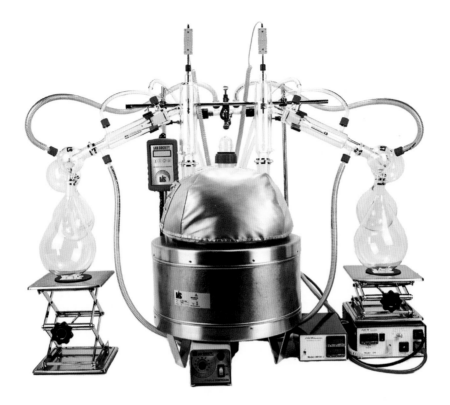

Distillers have traditionally been used in the alcohol industry, but for decades have also been used in cannabis processing, using alcohol as a solvent. Lab Society's Short Path Distillation Unit increases throughput, creating higher potency distilled oil. All of Lab Society's distillation kits include temperature controllers, termperature monitors and vacuum monitors for complete process control, as well as automation/data logging features.

DISTILLATION — FROM MOONSHINE TO MARY JANE

Unlike the chemical reaction behind solvent extraction, distillation is a physical separation and purification process that exploits the different respective boiling points of multiple components in the same mixture. Specifically, it allows for the removal of nonvolatile solids from volatile liquid, for example, removing salt from ocean water and distilling fresh water. It can also be used to isolate two volatile liquids, provided their respective boiling points are far enough apart, but more on that shortly.

Distillation has countless applications in human life but is largely associated with the purification of fermented ethanol into high-proof spirits for industrial or recreational purposes. Ethanol distillation involves heating a low-concentration mixture of ethanol and water, the product of fermentation, then collecting the resulting ethanol-rich steam. It goes to a condenser, which cools it and converts it back to a liquid, and voilà, distilled ethanol.

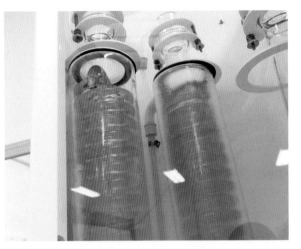

Alcohol steam is drawn away from the condenser, converting it back to liquid ethanol that is collected for reuse at LEVEL. This is done in the final steps after crude has been processed and winterized. Photo: Ed Rosenthal

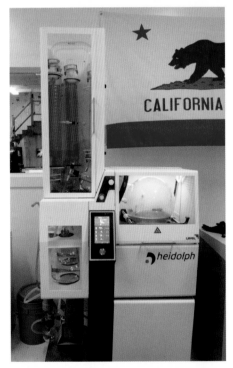

Commercial 20 L rotary evaporator at LEVEL. Ready to reclaim the last of the ethanol before final pass on the wiped film distillation unit.

The reason this process works is simple: The boiling point of water is 212°F, but the boiling point of ethanol is only 173.1°F. So when you heat the mixture at a temperature above 173.1°F, but under 212°F, the ethanol is selectively targeted, leaving most of the water behind. We stress most because ethanol is what's known as an azeotrope, the name for a mixture containing two liquids that share a single vaporization point at a given proportion.

"Pure" distilled ethanol still contains some water, even in its vapor state. In fact, we know exactly how much water because there's a natural "ceiling" on the potency of distilled ethanol without mechanical or chemical augmentation. Ever wonder why the maximum alcohol content of Everclear grain alcohol available is 190 proof? Why not 200 proof? Because it's physically impossible to exceed 190 proof through simple distillation: The purest ethanol achievable through just distillation is 95.57%. Further distillation at this potency will have no effect because the concentration of both the vapor and the liquid are equal.

To produce "molecular biology grade" ethanol, another hydrocarbon such as heptane or cyclo-hexane is added to augment the azeotrope and allow for more effective separation. Water and ethanol are both fractions, so there are physical limits on how "pure" their isolation can be through distillation.

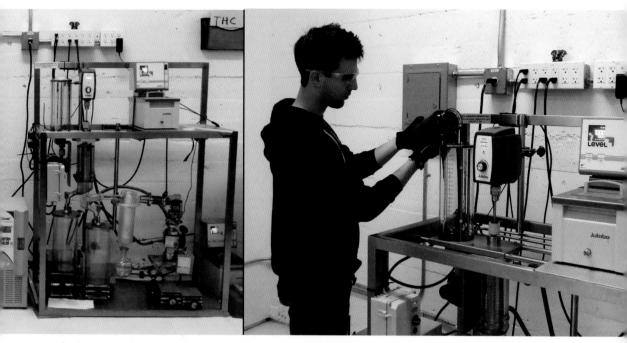

Left: Commercial-sized fractional distillation set-up at Level Labs.
Right: Flip Senn of Level Labs pouring crude oil into the fractional distillation machine.
Photos: Darcy Thompson

The term *fractional distillation* is used when multiple fractions are targeted from the same source material. You don't have to look far to find the result of fractional distillation in everyday life; you can see it in anything created with petroleum, which starts as crude oil that is refined into different products through industrial-scale fractional distillation. The science is simple: Gasoline has a higher boiling point than diesel fuel, but they're both present in crude oil. So by heating oil and capturing the vapors from these different fractions, a refinery can separate out all the useful products from a batch of crude — from the highly volatile "refinery gasses" and combustion fuels, which collect at the top of the fractionating column, down (literally) to the more or less inert asphalt sediments at the bottom of the column, with everything from gasoline to candle wax to petroleum jelly collected at points in between.

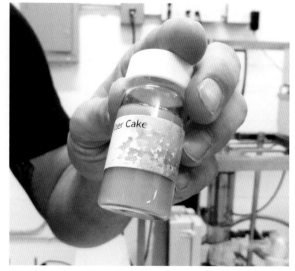

An example of waste material after a run at Level Labs. Photo: Darcy Thompson

A small fractionater can be used in a laboratory setup, but fractional distillation can also be achieved using a short-path setup with the addition of an extra condenser. Short-path distillation offers a slightly less complicated setup than a fractionater, but one that still can provide massive benefits to an extractor looking to refine a batch of BHO with less than desirable aesthetics and traits.

SIMPLE, SHORT PATH, FRACTIONAL — WHAT DOES IT MEAN?

To recap, simple distillation is used to remove nonvolatile solids from volatile liquids or to separate volatile liquids with boiling points more than 25°C apart; the process is generally done at regular atmospheric pressure. Short-path distillation, as the name implies, utilizes a very short pathway to reduce the amount of product that is lost through contact with equipment surfaces. The use of high pressure allows for distillation at lower temperatures. Fractional distillation is used when the boiling points of the fractions being targeted are less than 25°C apart.

There is a distinction between short-path and fractional distillation, but the separation of fractions from raw oil can be achieved using a short-path distillation setup in multiple passes. The value of fractional distillation is that it achieves in a single pass what it takes multiple passes to achieve with simple distillation.

Thin, or wiped-film, distillation dates to 1955, with the U.S. Navy's work to provide fresh water for submerged submarines. Primarily used to purify drinking water, this technique proves an interesting upgrade for a cannabis still. Specifically, it upgrades the heating and stirring element of traditional still setups. Instead of a large swirling vessel, a jacketed assembly with a wiper at the top is used. This wiper spreads the liquid crude in a very thin layer in an attempt to further increase potency and yields.

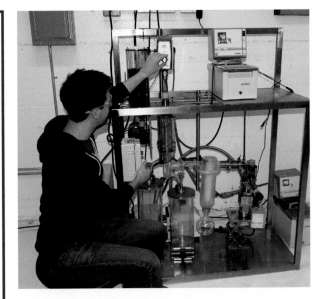

Flip Senn adjusting the vacuum pump and turning on the system after he loaded the crude oil. Notice how the three fractions at the bottom are already separating. Residue is collected in cylinder on the left and cannabinoids are collected in the center vessel. There right is a secondary pump, that is more refined of a pull on the far right.

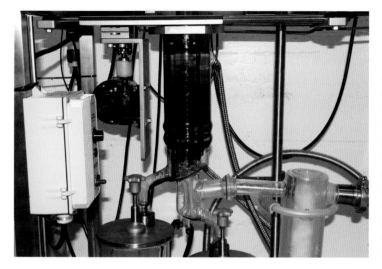

Gravity pulls the oil down, and the blades turning around the coil wipe the cannabis to four millimeters. This distills the oil over a very short distance and, as the gas evaporates and condenses onto the coil, the different fractions are made.
Photo: Ed Rosenthal

DISTILLING CANNABIS OIL

There are a number of parallels between liquor distillation and cannabis oil distillation, making it an excellent starting point for those wholly unfamiliar with the concept as it relates to cannabis. First and foremost, distillation is a secondary process that refines material extracted through some other method. When distilling bourbon whiskey, one starts by making a "mash," a concoction of water and grains that ferments, creating a mixture with a relatively low alcohol content. Similarly, when distilling "clear" distillate, you start with the product of solvent extraction — usually BHO, CO_2, or ethanol extract, which is distilled to further refine the THC fraction.

In whiskey distillation the mash is the product of fermentation; in cannabis distillation the "mash" is the product of a previous (often hydrocarbon) extraction process.

Like solvent extraction, fractional distillation is an industrial process that requires relatively expensive equipment, but as we've just covered, the organic chemistry at play is not particularly advanced. With a safe laboratory setup and a working understanding of the process, you can take subpar BHO, CO_2, or any other concentrate and separate out highly desirable elements, like specific terpenes and crystalline CBDa or THCa. Distillate can also be produced "from scratch" using buds or trim, without the intermediate step of making shatter or wax, but most producers do not use this approach because of the widespread availability of cheap, cannabinoid rich "crude" oil.

When applied to cannabis, the science of fractional distillation is the same as with petroleum products, but at a much smaller scale and using a different source material; cannabis "oleo resin," a broad term that encompasses all next-generation extracts that can be distilled. Instead of fuels and oils, fractional distillation of cannabis is targeting the usual suspects — terpenes and cannabinoids — but with a razor focus. Where solvent extraction removes and concentrates the terpenes and cannabinoids from raw flower, fractional distillation takes the concentrated cannabis resin created by solvent extraction and targets individual fractions. When performed properly, this process can create large crystals of solid THCa or CBDa with purity exceeding 99%. This process can also be used to isolate specific terpenes, which can be added back to the solids or used to flavor other products.

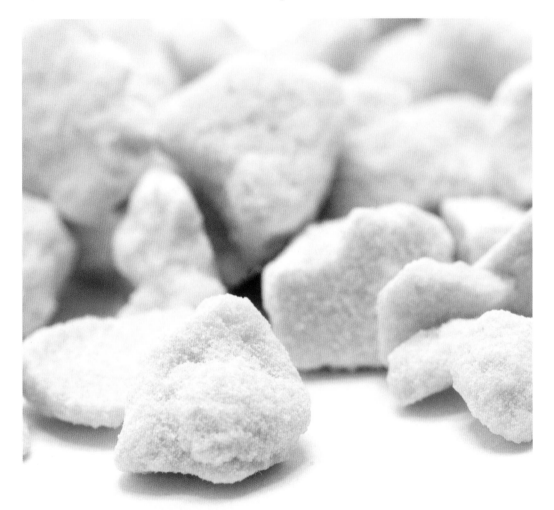

CBD isolate from Harmony Extracts

Theoretically, fractional distillation can be used to isolate any compound present in your starting material. Practically speaking, there are really only three salable products you can create using this process: crystalline THCa, crystalline CBDa, and terpenes. There are companies who isolate CBN, but mostly as an experimental novelty. There is no marked demand for any crystalline cannabinoids other than THC and CBD, but like all things related to cannabis extraction, that can change at any time.

PREPARING FOR FRACTIONAL DISTILLATION

Before you get down to the actual distillation process, you need to prepare your material, which means winterization. We cover the process of winterization in our "BHO" chapter, but here's a basic refresher: Starting material is combined with pure ethanol, heated and stirred until it fully dissolves into an alcohol solution. The solution is then placed in a freezer for 24 hours, where it freezes and causes separation of the residual lipids from the cannabinoids — terpenes are destroyed by the heat, so if you're trying to preserve them, they need to be extracted before winterization. The last step is mechanical filtration, which is achieved using a funnel and filter paper.

Once the oil has been winterized, it's sometimes mixed with other hydrocarbons and filtered through activated carbon or diatomaceous earth, but generally speaking, after winterization, it's time to begin distillation. Short-path distillation has several steps, but one of the most important is a thorough cleaning of the entire system including all hoses. You must use fresh vacuum pump oil every time.

Before you set up your apparatus, you need to double-check all of the glass components for any chips or cracks. If you find any, replace the damaged component before proceeding. NEVER use damaged lab equipment for any reason.

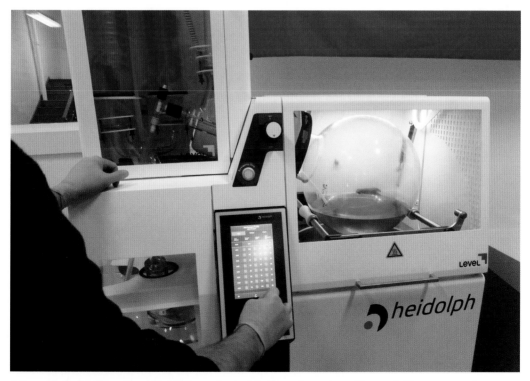

After winterization, the oil still has alcohol in it and must go through the process to remove the ethanol. Level Labs
Photo: Darcy Thompson

THE MATERIALS

Short-path distillation requires basic laboratory apparatus. To perform simple distillation, you will need the following:

- Laboratory heating mantle or a stirring hot plate
- Warm water bath
- Round bottom flask with magnetic stir bar
- Condenser adaptor
- Circulated chiller
- Thermometer adapter
- Thermometer
- Round bottom receiving flask
- Vacuum pump

THE PROCESS

1. **Check all glassware fittings and appliances for damage and cleanliness.**
   Every component of the distillation system should be thoroughly cleaned and inspected after and before each run. Under no circumstances should a cracked or otherwise damaged flask or fitting be used. If any part of your distillation system is dirty, clean it. If any part is broken, replace it. Do not proceed until all components are pristine.

2. **Assemble system, making sure all fittings are secured and all electrical components are plugged in and functional.**
   Fractional distillation will use the same setup as short-path distillation, but with the addition of an extra condenser — one vertical, the other horizontal. Condensers require "packing" to create surface area for condensation and reevaporation. There are many different types of packing, including metal rings and rods.

   It's very easy to overpack the column, and that tends to flood the column because the condensation will form a liquid plug. You should be able to see light through your packed condenser.

3. **Put on proper protective equipment**
   This step cannot be overstated. There's nothing uniquely dangerous about fractional distillation versus other forms of chemical extraction, but any chemical process entails some inherent hazards. The most skilled and experienced chemists can and do experience laboratory accidents, so it's absolutely crucial that proper eye and skin protection be used at all times to minimize the potential for injury.

4. **Bring the mantle to around 100°C and pull the still into its pressur-**

ized state with the vacuum to remove any excess moisture or invisible contaminants. Observe the condenser to make sure it's working and cooling properly. Air bubbles in the condenser indicate a leaky fitting. Run the chiller around 40°C.

5. **Load the product to be extracted into the flask that sits in your mantle. There's usually a sideport for this, and a metal funnel can help a lot.** The thermometer bulb needs to be level with the exit point from the boiling flask to the condenser — lower or higher orientation relative to the condenser exit will produce an artificially high or low temperature, respectively.

6. **Bring the mantle to around 190°C. There should be a consistent rolling boil in the product.** The use of a magnetic stir bar is absolutely crucial to avoid "bumping," a potentially lethal phenomenon that occurs when a large bubble of vapor forms in a confined, superheated solution and erupts from the opening in the container or even shatters it completely. This presents numerous opportunities for serious injury or worse, and can be easily avoided by using a magnetic stir bar, which will create a vortex in the fluid that prevents the formation of any large bubbles.

   The head may show some reflux of volatile compounds. Watch for a steady grip to form in the collection vessel. As you slowly raise the temperature, you will be separating a fraction. It flows from the head in a path to the collection vessel. The head should be around 123°C and rising.

7. **Observe mantle temperatures as they rise.** Terpenes will begin to collect in the cold trap as the temperature rises. Around 220°C a relatively high volume should be moving through the still. A common set point with short-path systems is 235°C. As you get close to this, the crude in your flask cooking on the mantle will darken up.

6. **After the mantle temperature rises to the set point or when you move out of fraction, you can turn the system off.** Open your release valve to depressurize and turn off your chiller pump and mantle. When the temperature of your system plateaus, that's the sign of a phase change, which means you're "in" a fraction. When the temperature begins to move meaningfully again, it's time to replace the collection flask and prepare for the next one.

7. **You can now remove your fractions.** Terpenes and a little THC will remain in your first fraction, as well as some terps in your cold trap, and the fractions of CBD in the remaining vessels.

8. **If desired, material from this first pass can be run again in a clean mantle for further refinement.**

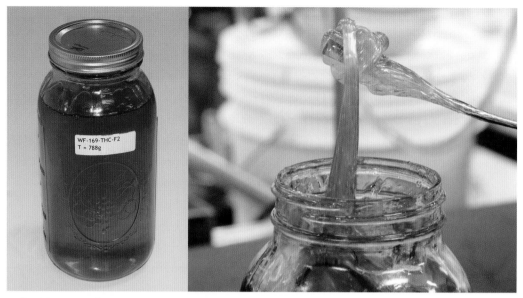

Left: Giant jar of distillate, 1800 grams.
Right: Distillate before packaging into vaporizer cartridges. Photos: Ed Rosenthal

At this point it is activated, highly concentrated cannabis extract, with a clear to slightly yellow appearance. A lot of times multiple passes on material are performed to improve the potency and appearance of the final product. It can be removed from the flask and packaged as a raw distillate, combined with terpenes and drawn into syringes or directly into vape cartridges. These distillations are highly desirable for the making of edibles as well as activated already and having very little flavor without re-added terpenes.

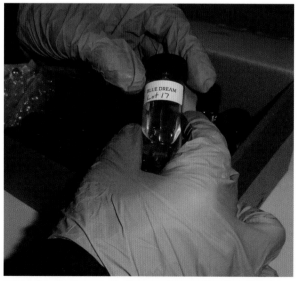

Blue dream terpenes from a box of bulk terpenes used in Level Labs vape cartridges.
Photo: Darcy Thompson

Further refinement leading to eventual isolation can include more purging through conventional means, the use of other hydrocarbons such as heptane or xylene, additional passes through a still, or more filtration.

As you can see, fractional distillation is far from the secretive sorcery many people perceive it to be. The cannabis plant is undeniably unique, but the processes being used to push its healing powers to their physical limits are the same ones standardized by nineteenth-century chemists. As the cannabis industry moves closer towards full legal legitimacy, the disparate tendrils of independent development and experimentation that brought us the products outlined in this book are coalescing into a unified understanding of the already established science.

The cannabis plant can take a very short or exceptionally long chemical journey these days. One path leads to drying, curing, and smoking. The other leads down a winding road of physical transformation: from plant matter to aqueous solution to oleo resin to distillate. Even then, the final destination of that distillate can be anything from immediate inhalation through a cartridge or a dab to further processing for use in topicals or edibles.

So while distillation may be the ultimate way to turn *Trash into Stash*, it also represents the cutting edge of the public's perception of cannabis. As cartridges and other distillate-based products continue to grow in popularity with THC and CBD consumers, there's no shortage of opportunity to create something using distillation that will be appreciated by many.

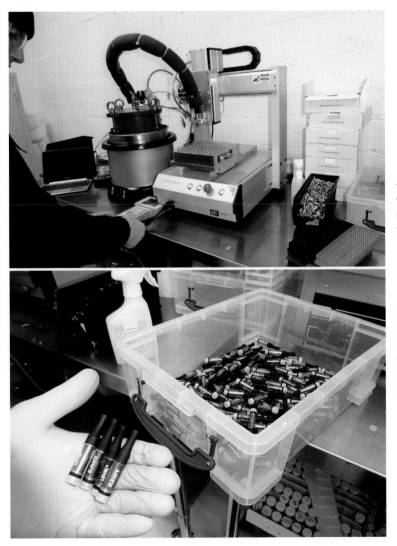

Jonathan Hoffman of LEVEL loads vape pen cartridges. Photo: Darcy Thompson

Finished vape pen cartridges ready to be packaged and distributed by LEVEL. Photo: Darcy Thompson

Alaska Thunder Fuck CO$_2$ extract at Heylo Cannabis Extracts in Seattle, WA
Photo: Kristin Angelo

CO$_2$ Extracts

When it comes to commercial-scale operations, CO$_2$ extraction is an efficient method for creating potent concentrates. Despite a relatively high start-up cost versus other methods, CO$_2$ enjoys widespread popularity, particularly with extractors producing oil to fill vape cartridges.

Unlike some of the other methods covered in this book, it can only be scaled down so much, meaning it's a less viable option for small producers. That said, there are several "white label" extractors who specialize in this process, meaning anyone with enough useable starting material can offer CO$_2$ products, so it's worth learning more about.

WHAT IS CO$_2$?

Carbon dioxide (CO$_2$) is a naturally occurring element; normally, it constitutes 0.039% of the air we breathe and is the central fuel of the photosynthesis process that plants use to stay alive.

Most of the time you can't see CO$_2$ because it's invisible as a gas, but many people are familiar with its solid form, a mainstay of several extraction methods: Dry ice. The defining feature of dry ice is that it sublimates directly from a solid to a gas, skipping over the messy liquid stage — this is where the "super critical" part comes in.

WHAT DO "SUBCRITICAL" AND "SUPERCRITICAL" MEAN?

CO_2 has no natural liquid state at atmospheric pressure. But at pressure greater than 5.1 standard atmosphere, it becomes a "supercritical fluid" that has physical characteristics of both gas and liquid, allowing it to effuse through material like gas while retaining the solvent properties of a liquid.

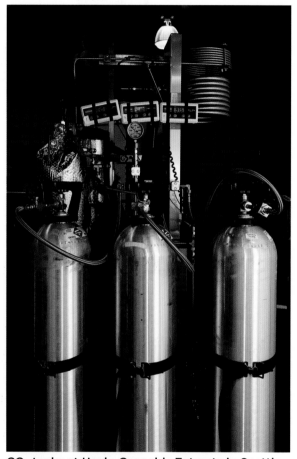

CO$_2$ tanks at Heylo Cannabis Extracts in Seattle, WA Photo: Kristin Angelo

"Supercritical" CO_2 extraction refers to extractions that occur beyond the "critical point" of carbon dioxide. Normally we think of CO_2 in gas, liquid, or solid form. But past CO_2's critical point, the molecule ceases to exist as a typical solid, liquid, or gas. Supercritical CO_2 looks like a very dense fog.

Supercritical fluid has no surface tension. It moves through vegetative material like a gas in a gaseous state and dissolves trichomes.

Carbon dioxide's supercritical state results from a combination of temperature and pressure. CO_2's supercritical range begins at 87°F (30°C) and 1070 psi. (By contrast, water goes supercritical at 700°F [371°C] and 4000 psi.) Supercritical fluid extraction (SFE) is usually performed at 800 to 5,000 psi.

"Subcritical" CO_2 extraction uses CO_2 in its liquid state, below its critical point. Pressure of between 800 and 1500 psi is applied to CO_2 at a temperature of 35°F (2°C)–55°F (13°C). The CO_2 liquid is pumped through plant material and it dissolves the oils and terpenes. Then the CO_2 is decompressed and returns to its gaseous state. The oils, consisting mostly of cannabinoids, terpenes, and waxes, precipitate and are collected on a nearby surface.

Supercritical fluid extraction has some advantages over subcritical (liquid) extraction. Supercritical fluids are faster extractors because of their low viscosities and high diffusiveness. CO_2 is pumped through the extracting material 3 to 10 times using supercritical, rather than 10 to 40 times using subcritical. Another advantage is that it can be used to select particular molecules for extraction by manipulating pressure and temperature.

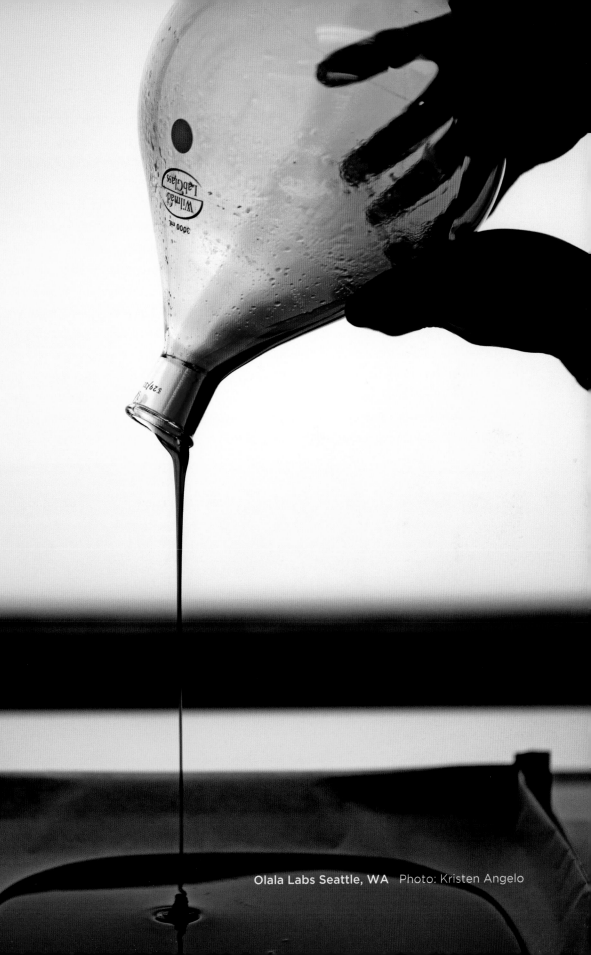

Olala Labs Seattle, WA   Photo: Kristen Angelo

The downside is supercritical fluid CO_2 reacts with moisture to form carbonic acid at pressures over 5000 psi, which can turns oils rancid. For this reason, all material used for CO_2 extractions must be less than 10% moisture..

Extract artists exploit the physical properties of liquid and supercritical CO_2 to extract and concentrate cannabinoids found on marijuana plants. The machines are expensive and require several days or more of training to operate, but have a number of advantages.

Large extraction companies are turning to CO_2 because of its proven efficiencies processing large amounts of leaf and trim. CO_2 extracts are four to five times as concentrated as the best buds, yet they can be inhaled without the irritation of smoking raw cannabis. They can also be used to make super potent edibles, topicals, smokables, and other marijuana-infused products. The best use of CO_2 on a commercial scale is the production of terpene rich vape pens.

CO_2 extraction is a relatively slow process, with super-critical CO_2 extraction taking 8–10 hours versus one hour or less for butane extraction. $SCCO_2$ extraction generally strips way more desirable terpenes than other methods. Many extractors still create very flavorful products using CO2, it just requires more fine-tuning of the process.

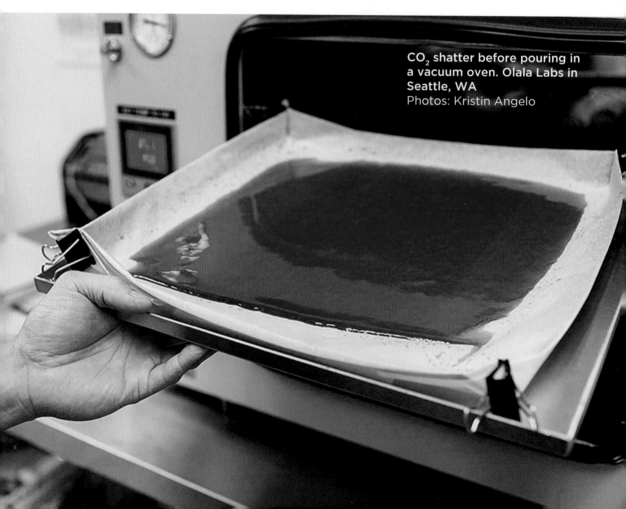

CO_2 shatter before pouring in a vacuum oven. Olala Labs in Seattle, WA
Photos: Kristin Angelo

A NOTE ON SCCO$_2$ EXTRACTION AND CONCENTRATE CONSUMPTION SAFETY

Proponents of CO$_2$ extraction argue that their process is superior to butane extraction.

The two primary arguments made in favor of CO$_2$ extraction speak to the producer and consumer respectively:

1. CO$_2$ extraction does not involve flammable solvents, so there is no physical risk associated with it.

2. CO$_2$ turns into water; such residual is "harmless" compared to residual hydrocarbons like butane.

Let's address the misconception behind argument one. It's true that CO$_2$ is not flammable, in fact, it's commonly used in fire extinguishers. But not all explosions are caused by combustion — the high pressure used in SCCO$_2$ can lead to explosions (more on that below), which can result in serious injury or death. Unlike butane extraction, which generally does not

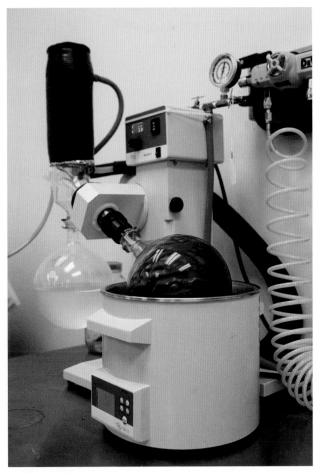

Rotary evaporator removing solvent

exceed pressures of 150 psi, CO$_2$ extraction routinely calls for pressure settings over 1,500 psi and can reach 8,700 psi.

Additionally, CO$_2$ is an asphyxiate, meaning that it displaces oxygen. Proper ventilation is crucial to safe CO$_2$ extraction: Always use a CO$_2$ detection mechanism to ensure high levels of CO$_2$ do not build up in your facility and kill you by forcing out oxygen.

In terms of the second argument, while supercritical CO$_2$ eliminates mold and other microbials during extraction, it has no impact on residual pesticides. The water left behind in CO$_2$ oil often contains pesticides used during cultivation. Corners can't be cut when it comes to sourcing starting material.

Loading cannabis into a CO_2 extractor at Heylo Cannabis Extracts in Seattle, WA
Photo: Kristin Angelo

EXPLOSION (YES, EXPLOSION) WARNING

CO$_2$ is nonflammable and nontoxic, but the extreme pressures that are utilized are dangerous unless contained by engineered and certified systems. Do not attempt to build your own CO$_2$ extractor because of the very real danger of explosion in materials not specifically engineered to withstand massive pressure. If you're not a licensed manufacturer of high-pressure equipment, don't risk your life and the lives of those around you by building a system that may fail and that can't be certified in the regulated market.

Wear safety glasses during extraction, although at higher pressures safety glasses will make little difference: When a 10,000 psi extractor fails, it creates an enormous bang like a shotgun going off and can damage anything in the immediate vicinity of the failing part. Technicians have lost their fingers trying to adjust a failing seal in the middle of a high-pressure extraction — don't risk it: If you suspect a failure, stop and depressurize the system.

OVERVIEW

Optimal CO$_2$ extraction involves using cool, pressurized carbon dioxide in either liquid or supercritical form to strip the cannabinoids and terpenes from the surface of the cannabis plant.

CO$_2$ is an extremely "tunable" solvent, which means different cannabinoids and terpenes can be targeted for extraction by altering the temperature and pressure settings.

CO$_2$'s boiling point is very low, which means the CO$_2$ will quickly evaporate from the extracted product with no need for a forced purging process. Once the CO$_2$ is purged from the solution, the plant's waxes, fats, lipids, and cannabinoids are left behind. The extraction process requires tanks of CO$_2$ and an extraction system engineered to withstand the low temperatures and high pressures used.

To begin the process, gas is liquefied and pumped through a pressure vessel packed with cannabis. The resulting mix is depressurized in a separator vessel, resulting in the cannabinoids, oils, waxes, and anything else in the solution falling out of the mix as the CO$_2$ flashes back to a gas, exits the vessel and is vented off, or is recovered and sent back to the pump in the case of a closed-loop system.

THE CO$_2$ EXTRACTION METHOD: WHAT'S NEEDED?

EQUIPMENT

- Plant material (frozen or fresh, cured, very dry, and trichome rich, cleaned of all debris)
- Liquid CO$_2$ cylinder with dip tube (a 50-pound cylinder goes for about $20; you'll need 75 pounds to extract 5 liters)

- CO_2 extractor (Eden Labs 5 liter, 2000 psi; Waters SFE 500 (Super Fluid Extractor).
- Industrial CO_2 pumps, rated anywhere from 5–10000 psi, .01–50 ml/min flow rate, +/-2% pressure accuracy; stainless steel fluid path
- Heater
- Chillers
- Condensing coil
- Cold gloves
- Pyrex dishes

CO_2 extract from Olala Labs, Seattle, WA
Photo: Kristin Angelo

TERMS OF EXTRACTION

Carbon dioxide extraction of cannabis fits into a broader practice of plant extraction that dates back hundreds of years. Plant extracts are used extensively in medicine, nutraceuticals, and the perfume industry. The industry breaks down plant extracts in to three general categories, each more refined: essential oils, concretes, and absolutes.

Essential Oils: An essential oil is a concentrated hydrophobic liquid containing the volatile aroma compounds and other "essential" molecules of a plant — including its lipids and, in the case of pot, its cannabinoids. Essential oils are obtained by pressure or steam, water, or dry distillation.

Concretes: Essential oil extracts made from hydrophobic solvent are called concretes and are a mixture of oil, waxes, resins, and other oil-soluble plant material, like THC. They can be hard, malleable, or viscous, depending on wax content.

Absolutes: Concretes treated with another solvent to remove their waxes and leave just the fragrant, essential oil are called absolutes. They're usually highly concentrated viscous liquids but can be solid or semisolid.

INTRODUCTION TO GEAR

Here are the basic components of a CO2 supercritical extractor (SFE machine) from beginning to end:

- CO$_2$ supply — your tanks of CO$_2$
- Cooling bath / heat exchanger — to ensure CO2 is in a liquid state when it goes to pump
- CO$_2$ pump — the heart of the system; receives liquid CO$_2$ at 750 psi and takes it to supercritical levels
- Heater / heat exchanger — used to raise pressurized CO$_2$ to supercritical temperatures
- Extraction vessel — where CO$_2$ and plant matter meet and extraction occurs
- Back-pressure regulator — reduces pressure, turning supercritical CO$_2$ back to a gas, causing precipitation of solutes
- Fraction collector / collection vessel — where precipitated solutes collect
- Vent — where CO$_2$ comes out of the system
- CO$_2$ condenser / chiller — used to reliquefy CO$_2$ for recycling

SYSTEM SETUP AND CHECKS

CO$_2$ extraction units range in size from desktop to industrial plants and need to be placed in a structure that has enough power and ventilation, ideally something like a mechanic's bay. Smaller systems run on 110V, but larger systems usually use 220V circuits. The pumps, heat exchangers, and other equipment generate heat and noise, so the space must be able to accommodate it.

Each equipment manufacturer's machines have their own procedures and techniques. For that reason, the equipment comes with comprehensive guides. Some manufacturers provide personal training on the use of their systems and process development, since the process can be quite complex.

You'll want to create a safety checklist and standard operating procedure based on the instructions from the manufacturer. As a general rule, make sure all seals are tight, but don't overtighten or cross-thread them.

EXTRACTION STEPS

After your system is all set up and you're trained on it, follow the basic extraction steps below.

1. Warm everything up: Start up the chiller and the heat exchangers. They need a bit of time to warm water or cool coolant to their set points. Bringing hundreds of pounds of stainless steel extraction equipment to its specific operating temperatures can take about an hour.
2. Load the extraction vessel with your prepared material and bolt secure the lid.
3. Pressure test the system for 15–20 minutes to make sure that there are no leaks. Keep a watchful eye on the gauges for sudden pressure drops or temperature changes.
4. Extract: Send liquid CO_2 through the pump, which raises its pressure between 800 and 5000 psi. The 80°F (27°C) heater makes the liquid go supercritical. The CO_2 mixes with the trim in the extraction vessel, dissolves the plant's oils, and flows out to the back-pressure regulator.
5. Precipitate: The back-pressure regulator takes the supercritical CO_2 solution from 5000+ psi to 350–900 psi, flashing it back to a gas and causing the essential oil to fall out.
6. Vent/Recirculate: CO_2 is then vented outside the building or sent to the compressor/chiller that reliquefies the CO_2 and sends it back to the beginning of the system. It can take 20 minutes up to 10 hours to fully extract from trim, depending on solvent throughput, process parameters, vessel size, and trim potency.
7. Depressurize the extraction vessel and open the drain valve (if the system has one) to receive the oil.
8. Clean: Run the system dry empty with CO_2 to clean it. Clean in-between different strains and as needed depending on system use.

CO$_2$ concentrate being removed
from the extraction equipment at
Olala Labs in Seattle, WA
Photo: Kristin Angelo

TIPS

You'll get more consistent results at the low end of the supercritical range. The higher you go in the supercritical range, the hotter and more soluble the CO_2 becomes, which can pull unwanted compounds such as chlorophyll. However, higher temperature and pressure can decrease run times, and chlorophyll can be avoided with proper methodology.

As gas drains from the CO_2 tank, it depressurizes and cools. This can create bubbles or voids in the line, which can cause flow problems. Prevent these bubbles by not using nearly empty CO_2 tanks. Use a scale to keep an eye on how much CO_2 is left in a tank. When it gets to a certain weight indicating that it's low, swap it out.

Keep the temperature in the extraction room at a consistent 65°F (18°C) to 72°F and keep humidity as low as possible. Don't extract in hot environments; the ambient heat will work its way into your system and sap your yield.

Purchase an American-made extractor. You're going to need the manufacturer's staff to train you, and you're going to be calling them when you run into problems or need replacement parts such as o-rings, etc.: An SFE machine is a very hands-on product.

The pump is the heart of the SFE system and must be designed to withstand operating pressures and temperatures for prolonged periods of time. Waters, Apeks, and Eden Labs sell appropriate pumps. The pump is the part of the system that is most likely to require servicing, and they can run tens of thousands of dollars. Broken pumps are the chief cause of downtime of some systems, particularly gas booster pumps. Prevent this by having a backup or replacement pump so the system can continue functioning while the pump is being serviced. You can also avoid considerable downtime by purchasing a system that utilizes a liquid pumping system such as Eden Labs or Waters.

You can reuse CO_2 2 to 4 times depending on the amount of oil in the start material. After a certain point the solvent becomes saturated with oil and will no longer pull oils from the plant material.

A compressor and chiller reliquefies CO_2, and charcoal microfilters scrub out the water and other impurities. Still, it will eventually have to be vented off. It's still suitable to use for enriching gardens with CO_2.

PURGING

With CO_2 you don't really have to purge, unless you're using a high amount of cosolvent, such as ethyl alcohol, which is used in some machines.

Raw CO_2 oil comes out of the drain valve bright red, yellow, orange, or amber. If it's green, chlorophyll has been extracted which most likely means one of five things is happening: the pressure is too high; the temperature is too high; the material is old, stale, or wet. Moisture changes the pH of CO_2, making it more acidic and polar. Acidic, polar solvents extract chlorophyll and other

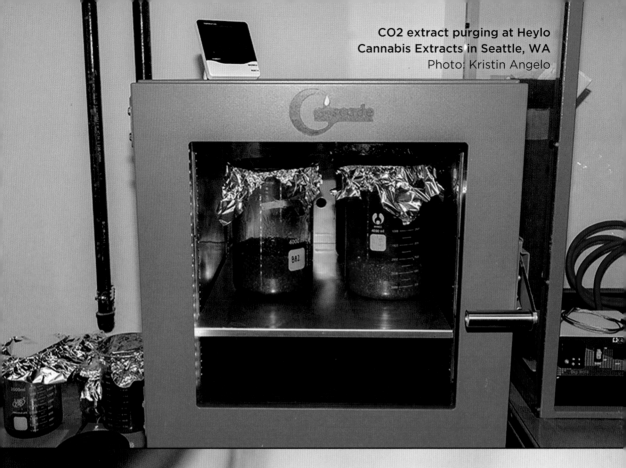

CO2 extract purging at Heylo Cannabis Extracts in Seattle, WA
Photo: Kristin Angelo

Muffin of raw oil from an intitial pull at Olala Labs, Seattle, WA
Photo: Kristin Angelo

undesired elements.

If used in an open system, the CO_2 evaporates to a gas from its supercritical or liquid state and returns to the atmosphere. Vent it outside or slowly in a grow room to avoid asphyxiation.

The process yields thick-varying viscosities of oil or "crumble" depending on strain and processing parameters. Whether the starting material was grown indoors or outdoors and the processing parameters can play a role in determining how much wax is in the raw oil.

When the paste extract is left sitting in the open air, it slowly settles into a blob, sort of like a bead of water on a hydrophobic surface, or into an oil-like consistency.

Commercial manufacturers sometimes add propylene glycol to the oil to make it runnier for flowing into pens and cartridges.

By changing the techniques, you can make different consistencies, such as a honeycomb-like crumble consistency or slow-flowing or hardened oils by dewaxing the material.

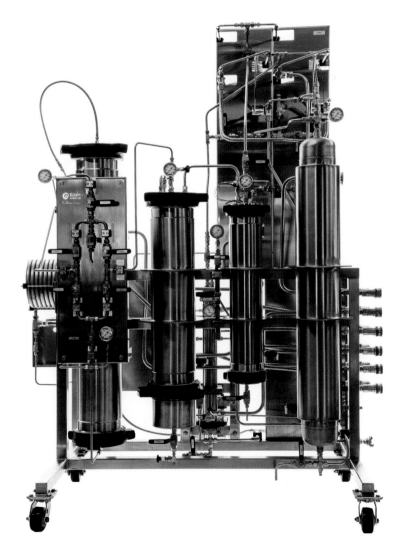

WINTERIZATION/DEWAXING

Winterization in chemistry refers to the removal of waxes from a solution, usually by means of cold temperature. There are several ways to dewax CO$_2$ oil in the depressurization stage of extraction. One way is to treat CO$_2$ oil with another solvent, usually alcohol, to dewax it. Winterization boosts THC levels from 50%–70% to 80%–90%, but the increase comes at the expense of terpenes, which are lost in the process.

DECARBOXYLATION

To use CO$_2$ concentrates in edibles, they must first be decarboxylated.

VARIATIONS

Strain, growing environment, harvest time, curing method and length, material preparation and batch size all play roles in the outcome of CO$_2$ extraction.

One strain may extract twice as fast as another strain. Strains also vary in yield, color of the oil, and consistency. Cannabinoid ratios play a role in solubility, color, taste, and smell. Using all buds, small nugs, trim, or a combination also results in different quality oils.

Keep variables to a minimum. To get a repeatable outcome, collect the data and track the entire process from material acquisition to packaging. Invest in a testing system to test each lot purchased and test the oil as it is processed. This will give you the intelligence you need to ensure your process parameters are optimal for that lot and the product desired. It's impossible to estimate process efficiencies without knowing how much oil is in the start material and how to best release it unless there is due diligence of testing and excellent record keeping.

Fully automated computerized systems like an Apeks or Waters CO$_2$ SFE machine reduce variability and produce more consistent oil compared to manual systems, but not all manufacturers recommend them.

STORAGE/PRESSING

CO$_2$ extracts should be refrigerated in a silicone or other stick-proof container. Oils stored at room temperature degrade and turn rancid because of carbonic acid. Long-term exposure to air or light also causes unwanted reactions with the active ingredients.

CO$_2$ oil or honeycomb — the two most common consistencies — do not need pressing. The trichome heads were already broken in the violent extraction process and the active compounds dissolved into the solution before being chilled out of it.

Left: A high-tech example of a closed-loop CO$_2$ extractor: Eden Labs' Hi-FloTM 20L Extraction System. Carbon Dioxide is a relatively safe, non-volatile extraction solvent. Some refer to this process as "solventless extraction."

Eden Labs

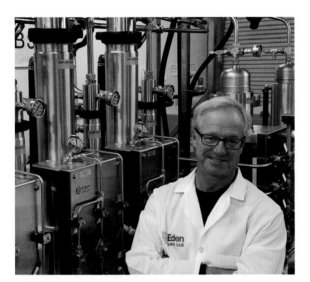

Eden Labs was founded in Ohio in 1994, and it's currently headquartered in Seattle, Washington, but it has deep roots in California's medical cannabis movement: After the passage of Proposition 215 in 1996, the company's signature Coldfinger™ ethanol extraction system became the first commercial-size cannabis extractor installed in a San Francisco dispensary.

Eden Labs founder Fritz Chess was a science journalist with an abiding interest in botanical medicine. His research into herbal medicine created and used by remote indigenous peoples sparked a curiosity about extracting botanical remedies using distillation and other contemporary technologies. That curiosity transformed into dedication, and producing a system for extracting healthy, natural products became his personal mission.

The Coldfinger™ system started as a radical redesign of the century-old soxhlet extractor, and during this same R&D period Fritz engineered and built the first supercritical CO_2 system optimized for heavy resinous oils — a revolutionary development in supercritical fluid extraction. The system was affordable and exceedingly easy to operate, allowing small businesses to access technology that was previously out of their reach.

Eden Lab's CEO, AC Braddock, joined the company in 2009; within three years, Eden was recognized by Inc.com as one of the "Top 10 Fastest Growing Women-Led Companies in Seattle." Braddock's leadership is guided by an unwavering belief in whole plant medical applications and a commitment to an ethical, holistic approach to business. Her keen eye for new trends, product placement, business strategy, and political involvement contribute to a vibrant corporate culture that's making waves nationally.

The force that animates Eden Labs is the same one that inspired its founding — curiosity. Eden's R&D team is constantly pushing the limits of innovation and chasing the leading edge of extraction technology. By engineering advanced systems that reliably produce high-grade products, Eden has distinguished itself as an industry leader and created a brand known for quality and customer success.

Thanks to that success, the demand for large, industrial-grade extraction systems has grown organically. Eden now offers supercritical fluid extraction units up to 6,000 liters and 500 gallons for ethanol in industries including nutraceuticals, flavorings, fragrances, biofuels, herbal medicines, and more.

But Eden Labs is more than just a technology and market leader in the world of botanical extraction tech: it's a legit "OG" of cannabis extraction. Whether you're chasing a single molecule or a blend of botanical essences, few companies offer the broad, product-specific knowledge and technological expertise needed to achieve your extraction goals.

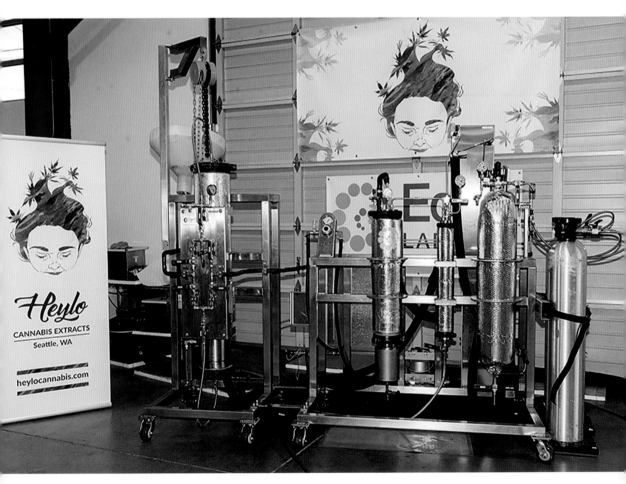

BAS Research

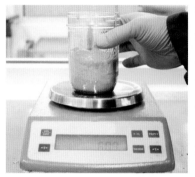

To truly grasp the mission and origin of BAS Research, you first need to understand the journey of Dr. Bao Le and his son Andrew, an autistic boy who has battled with seizures and night terrors for most of his young life. After Le started researching the potential of CBD and THC to help alleviate his son's symptoms, he soon decided to dedicate his life to finding safe and holistic treatment alternatives for Andrew and others in his position.

However, when he started looking for trusted sources of cannabis oil, Le found it difficult to secure a reliable source for lab-tested oils that were completely free of pesticides and other dangerous contaminants. So instead of continuing this fruitless search, Le decided to launch an extraction and manufacturing company of his own, founded with the goal of developing sound scientific methods to consistently and safely extract essential oils from the cannabis plant

Using the Pharmaceutical, Nutraceutical and Agricultural industries as a model, BAS Research set out to create best practices and standard operating procedures (SOP's) for its cannabis extraction processes. The company is also committed to fighting the negative social stigma associated with cannabis, by demonstrating that cannabis can be processed with safe, natural methods.

Le's hard work paid off when BAS Research received one of the first licenses to manufacture from the city of Berkeley in 2016. Later that year the company secured a strategic partnership with Montel Williams and his company, Lenitiv Labs. Williams was diagnosed with Multiple Sclerosis (MS) in 1999 and has used cannabis products ever since as a medication to manage the disease's symptoms.

As more and more cannabis products require cannabis oil as a fundamental ingredient, BAS Research's oils can now be found in wide range of cannabis medicine in the marketplace, from vape cartridges to tinctures and topical creams. Through its unique production process, BAS is able to customize oil blends and other extracts to the specific needs of its customers. For instance, an edibles company may require an odorless tasteless oil to blend into its products, while a vape cartridge supplier might want quite the opposite – a custom, flavorful blend of natural cannabis

phytomaterials that incorporates flavors from multiple strains.

Extraction science plays a fundamental role in harvesting components of the cannabis oils from the plants. Solubilities of the various molecules in another material, such as supercritical carbon dioxide (CO_2), determine the composition of the different extracts the company produces. To arrive at the best extraction methods for different strains, BAS technicians map the characteristics of each extract as the temperature and pressure are carefully manipulated for set periods of time.

Some of the company's more popular products include a Winterized Amber Oil, which is a cannabinoid-rich CO_2 extract that is refined into a translucent amber colored oil of medium viscosity and high potency through a careful removal of fats, lipids, and waxes. Primarily used for vape technologies, it can be produced in strain-specific, terpene-enriched variations and is also available as THC or CBD-dominant. The Distilled Clear Oil is a transparent and lightly golden concentrate that is decarboxylated and can be used directly as a plain distillate or be reintroduced to its terpenes for the full effect of the cannabis entourage.

Regardless of the end product, BAS Research always has its fundamental values in mind as it manufactures extracts.

"CBD and THC saved my son," says Le. "Without it he has days of not being able to sleep when his night terrors affect him. Having experienced first-hand how CBD and THC is helping my son, I encourage everyone to research the benefits and effects of cannabis with an open mind."

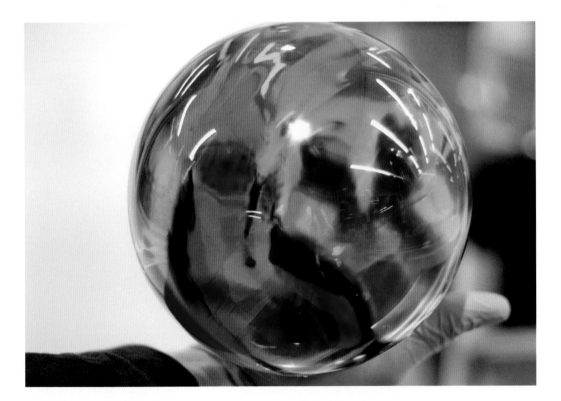

Sour HS 70u hash by Nikka T
Photo: Nikka T

CHAPTER 7

Hash to the Future

From Dry Sift to Machine Hash

Kief, also known as "Dry Sift," is composed of the unpressed glands scraped from dried mature flowers and leaves using a screen. It is very popular because it is easily gleaned from leaves and trim.

Kief is the easiest marijuana product you can make. Tiny resin-filled glands cover the buds and leaves. These tiny stalked glands, known as trichomes, are the only part of the plant that contain significant amounts of cannabinoids, such as THC and CBD, as well as the pungent terpenes that give each marijuana strain its distinctive aroma, taste, and medical and psycho-active qualities. Making kief consists of collecting those trichomes. There are a number of techniques for separating them from the plant material and sorting them.

Kief can be smoked just as it is collected; you can add the kief to your pipe without further processing or preparation. It is often pressed to make hash. It can also be used to produce tinctures or cooking ingredients. Those uses are discussed in their respective chapters. This chapter explains various screening techniques to produce kief, as well as methods using ice, dry ice or CO_2 to enhance the process.

Because kief is so easy to collect from dried cannabis it is one of the oldest marijuana preparations and is known in many corners of the world. Alternatively spelled as *kif, kief, kef,* or *kiff,* the word appears in many languages. The origin of the word is the Arabic *kayf,* which means well-being or pleasure. The term was historically used in Morocco and elsewhere to mean a mixture of marijuana and tobacco, not unlike modern-day spliffs or blunts, though it was typically smoked using hookahs. In Amsterdam and other parts of Europe, kief is sometimes called pollen or polm, and many of the screens and devices used to separate kief from other plant material are called pollen screens or pollen sifters.

The marijuana plant produces three basic types of resin-rich glands that grow to different sizes expressed in microns or micrometers, which is a metric measurement equal to one millionth of a meter. Marijuana glands or trichomes range from as small as 15 microns to as large as 500 microns. That lets you easily separate the different glands by using screens of corresponding sizes.

The bulbous glands are the smallest, ranging from 10 to 15 microns. These tiniest glands perch atop equally tiny one-cell stalks that cover the leaves of vegetative plants.

The capitate-sessile glands are the middle size, ranging from 25 to100 microns, and are more numerous than the bulbous glands. "Capitate" means globular, and that's what they look like—spherical globs of resin that lay on the leaf and flower surfaces.

Capitate-stalked glands are the ones most visible on the buds of mature, flowering marijuana plants, as these rich resin balls are the largest at 150–500 microns, and they sit high on stalks that can reach 500 microns. These are the glands that hold most of the cannabinoids and terpenes and are found most abundantly on the upper leaves, flowers, and bracts (the tiny leaves surrounding the flowers) of unfertilized female plants. These are the glands that are captured to make kief.

The maturity of the plant and its variety and environmental conditions all affect gland size. For instance, many Moroccan varieties may have glands that are under 80 microns. Many sativa varieties also have small glands. "Hash plant" varieties often have glands that are 120 microns or larger. Most sinsemilla is in the mid-range, between 80 and 110 microns.

To give you a sense of these sizes, a human hair is about 70 microns or a bit more; the finest beach sand is 100 microns; playground sand is roughly 250 microns and the eye of a needle is more than 1200 microns.

To measure the size of the glands with precision use a microscope and a slide with a micron scale etched on it. Some microscopes come equipped with a scale called a reticule built into one of the eyepieces to measure microns. Count the number of hash marks the gland spans and multiply by the conversion factor for the magnification power.

HOW KIEF SCREENING WORKS

THC and other cannabinoids and terpenes are concentrated in glands that cover many parts of the marijuana plant, but they're concentrated in the upper leaves, flowers, and flower bracts of unfertilized female plants. They are also found on the seed covering and surrounding areas of pollinated plants. Screening cured plant material is one of the easiest ways to rescue these glands for use.

There are several different ways to prepare the plant material for screening or sifting. In countries close to the 30th parallel, such as Nepal, Afghanistan, and Lebanon, small amounts of kief have traditionally been made using a silk scarf stretched tightly over a bowl. Dried marijuana, frequently cured for as long as six months, is rubbed on the taut silk cloth. The cloth's fine weave allows the small glands to pass through to the bowl, leaving the vegetative material on top. Silk scarves are still used in parts of the world, but the nylon or metal mesh screens used for printing (still often called silk screens) are more durable and come in a variety of dimensions and mesh sizes.

One of the simplest methods of making kief is by gently rubbing the plant material over a fine screen. The size of the openings in the screen determines which size glands and how much residual plant material will make it through. The vigor used in rubbing the material on the screen has a profound effect on the quality of the final product. Different grades of kief are produced by varying the amount of time the material is sifted, the screen's gauge, and the pressure used. Sifting the same material a few times yields more kief, but each sift results in a

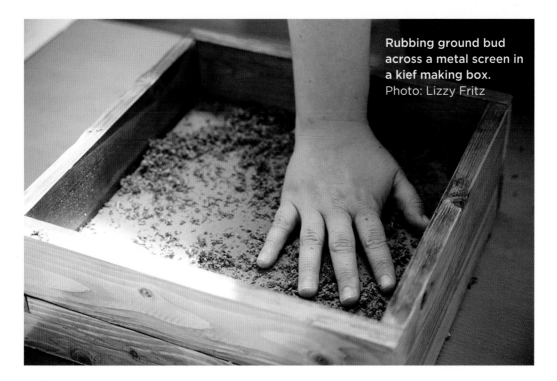

Rubbing ground bud across a metal screen in a kief making box.
Photo: Lizzy Fritz

higher proportion of plant matter mixed with the glands. Kief color ranges from golden white for the purest kief to a greenish gold. The greener it is the more plant material it contains.

Kief or pollen-sifting boxes are good tools for making small amounts; they can be as simple as wooden stash boxes with a screen above a pullout drawer that catches the glands that fall off your weed in normal handling. Other boxes are made specifically to capture different grades of kief, separating the glands from the vegetation by shaking it. Overvigorous shaking or rubbing is counterproductive because too much vegetation is collected, lowering the quality. Use cold material. Freezing makes it crisp so the glands break free easier.

Some larger sifters are automated, much like a paint mixer, so you can add the material, flip a switch, and let the sifter do the work.

Compact DIY solutions are inexpensive and easy to make from screens used for printing T-shirts and posters. All you need is the proper screen, a frame to stretch it on, and a smooth hard surface such as glass or metal to collect the kief.

Printing screens made of nylon, polyester, or metal are available at art supply stores or online. The mesh sizes are typically described in terms of the number of threads per inch, so a higher number is a finer screen. Meshes range from around 40 to 400, with 110 and 156 being the most common for printing T-shirts. Screen mesh can be purchased pre-stretched in aluminum or wood frames or as rolls or sheets.

GLANDS AND SCREENS: A GUIDE

Matching screen size to gland size is important for maximizing your kief yield. Most marijuana glands are typically between 75 to 125 microns or micrometers, though they vary based on the type of gland, the maturity of the plant, and other factors. Mesh screens are usually sized by a "mesh" measurement that indicates how many strands of wire or nylon it has for every inch of material. Detailed mesh-to-micron conversion charts can be found online, but the chart below shows common mesh sizes and the micron size of the openings between strands. (LPI stands for lines per inch.) Kief sifting generally works best with screens between 100 and 130 microns. Plants with larger crystals need a screen of 150 microns to capture the glands. Screens in the range of 100-150 lines per inch usually work well. But not all

Inches	LPI	Microns	Millimeters
0.0021	270	53	0.053
0.0024	230	63	0.063
0.0029	200	74	0.074
0.0035	170	88	0.088
0.0041	140	105	0.105
0.0049	120	125	0.125
0.0059	100	149	0.149
0.0070	80	177	0.177

mesh sizes are created equal. The size of the openings varies based on the diameter of the strands. Screens made of nylon, polyester, or stainless steel have different strand diameters at any particular mesh size, and finer mesh screens use strands of smaller diameters. Stainless steel screens are the most durable and don't shed. Plastic and nylon screens should be replaced periodically because they shed strands as they age and wear.

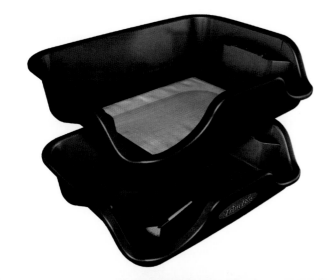

Left: The Trimbin by Harvest More is sturdy, ergonomic, and meant to sit on the user's lap. Collect kief with the 150 micron stainless steel screen while you prep your bud.

Below: Save time on the debudding process with the Official DeBud-der™ Bucket Lid that allows you to easily debud your harvest, removing the stems and catching the buds in a standard bucket.

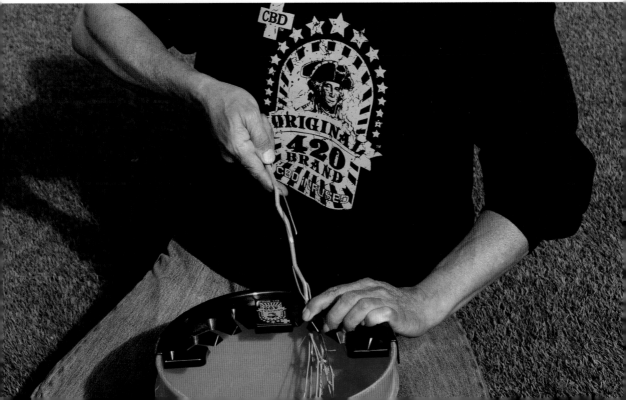

Isolating the resin glands that contain the flavors and effects of cannabis from the largely inert plant material is far from a new idea. The old methods of concentration are used to create hashish, often called hash. The practice began millennia ago, probably in Asia near the Hindu Kush region. But there is a rich historical tradition of cannabis extraction across Asia, the Middle East and North Africa, home to historical hash capitals including India, Nepal, Afghanistan, Pakistan, Lebanon, and Morocco.

Perhaps the oldest way of making hash is hand-rubbing fresh cannabis plants and collecting the resin that accumulates on your fingers and palms, then rolling it into balls or coils. This is called charas. The resulting product is prized globally and the legends of its unique potency still attract travelers to the northern Himalayas, where it's made on a large scale. The yields from charas are low. It requires much more material and far more labor than other methods. The process can produce extremely high-quality hash, but because the resin is collected fresh from the plant and is still very sticky, it is pressed by working it with palms and fingers into a ball or patty until it dries a bit.

Another classic method of hash production involves suspending dried cannabis plants over tarps and collecting the glands that fall naturally and pressing them into hashish. Many contemporary methods for "dry sifting" hash still exist, ranging in complexity from small boxes lined with screens for collecting kief from a personal use stash, to mechanical tumblers that agitate the cannabis and screen out the glands.

The techniques outlined in this chapter can all trace their lineage directly to hash makers of antiquity, because the core physical principles are unchanging; manually removing the resin glands using cold and physical agitation, then concentrating the resin using heat, pressure, and time.

DRY ICE KIEF — THE MANUAL METHOD

Perhaps the cheapest, simplest way to concentrate cannabinoids is also one of the newest. Since 2009, hash makers have been turning to dry ice — which is frozen carbon dioxide—to yield an impressive amount of kief. Dry ice is the fastest way to turn trash into gold. Manual dry ice sieving is very inexpensive to set up, results in very little mess or cleanup, and doesn't involve explosive chemicals like BHO, or require expensive machinery like CO_2 and other methods of extraction.

One-Minute Dry Ice Kief is very smooth and contains a lot of terpenes because it's made cold and not mixed with anything, even water, preserving the natural terpenes. It has very little vegetation so you're inhaling only gland products.

EQUIPMENT
- Cannabis (1 ounce, dry trim or fresh frozen)
- Bubble Bags (durable 160- and 220-micron water bubble bags)

Dry ice kief from Ed Rosenthal's homegrown blue dream. Photo: Lizzy Fritz

- 5-gallon bucket
- Clean, sanitary surface area — at least four feet long
- Collection tool (such as a plastic scraper)
- Dry ice — 3 pounds, broken up into small pieces

METHOD

Manual dry ice sieving uses the -106°F (-76°C) temperature of dry ice to freeze the waxy stalks of the trichomes, making them brittle enough to snap off during agitation. The snapped glands then fall through the 160- or 220-micron bag onto a surface and are collected.

First, designate a clean, sanitary, indoor space with a clean surface. Sanitary conditions are important; you don't want to find dog hair or other contaminants in the final product. Set up a large table in the clean room and cover it with some parchment paper. Place trim or ground bud in the bucket. Add dry ice. Tightly affix the 160-micron bubble bag over the top of the bucket using large rubber bands so that when you eventually turn the bucket upside down, the dry ice and trim fall onto the screen.

Pick up the bucket and gently shake to help distribute the cold. After a minute, turn the bucket upside down and hold it over the parchment paper. The dry ice and trim fall to the bottom of the bag.

Lightly shake the dry ice and trim mix up and down, moving longitudinally along the surface of the table so the falling kief creates a trail several feet long.

As you do this, the kief dust will fall down from the bag onto the paper, amid little puffs of evaporating carbon dioxide. Keep shaking for 30 seconds to sieve the trichomes through the filter. You will notice that the first glands are a pale golden-yellow and that as the process continues, the trail of glands gets greener because more vegetative material is in the mix. The first material to fall, the golden gland, is the highest quality.

Use a scraper to collect the kief, which (should smell phenomenal) and store it in a clean glass jar.

Repeat the process using the 220-micron bag and collect the kief. One ounce of dried sugar leaf trim yields about four grams of kief at 160 microns, and six more lower-grade grams of kief at 220 microns.

TIPS

- Dry ice sieving kief sends weed dust everywhere unless the bucket bottom, is kept close to the table surface.
- Avoid working in areas with breezes or running fans.
- Use thinner chunks of dry ice and less agitation for purer kief.
- Use quality nylon mesh bubble bags; plastic mesh bags degrade under the brutal cold of the dry ice.
- If you're making your own device, use stainless steel mesh rather than nylon. The nylon wears and chips when it's frozen by the dry ice. Stainless steel lasts indefinitely.
- You can use either dried or fresh-frozen trim. Both kief out nicely, and the latter contains more terpenes.

HOW TO MAKE DRY ICE KIEF (HASH) — STEP BY STEP

Place 4 ounces brittle dry bud in a 5-gallon bucket.

1. Add 3 pounds of dry ice — it should be ice cube size or smaller. Ideally the dry ice should be placed both under and on top of the grass — sandwiching the material. Let the mixture cool for 2 minutes.
2. Place a 220-mesh screen bag over the bucket top.
3. Turn the bucket upside down and start shaking it vigorously, moving down a 6- or 8-foot table or countertop in about 2 minutes.

4. The powder changes color from a golden to a greenish tint over the table length — golden is the purest, highest quality. The powder was separated into higher- and lower-quality portions.

5. The two piles — they are ready to be smoked, pressed, or used in recipes.

6. A pile of fine, blonde, dry ice hash beckons all to take a toke.

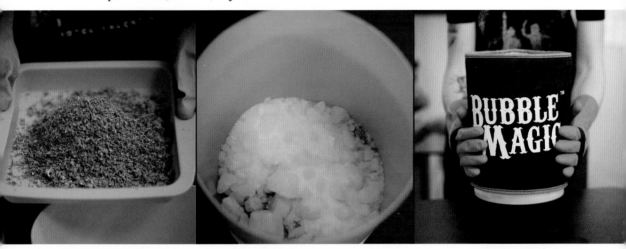

Ground blue dream buds.

Dry ice and cannabis in a bucket, chilling before it is flipped over a screen.

The screen placed over the bucket.

Dry ice hash passes through the screen in a golden shower.
Photos: Lizzy Fritz

Bubble hash magnified.
Photo: Marcus Bubbleman

WATER HASH 101

Water hash is another favorite method of making concentrates employed all over the world. Its name comes from the water process used to collect glands from the trim, leaf, and buds. On a fundamental level, the process works because cannabinoids are not water soluble, meaning that the desired resins are not damaged by contact with water and ice.

Water hash can be smoked as loose, granular resin or pressed into traditional hashish: High-quality loose hash can easily be pressed into hashish using nothing more than the palm of one hand and some light, brisk friction, applied using the thumb of the other hand. Loose or pressed, many people are still enthralled by the unique, full-spectrum experience of this potent natural product.

Water hash can be made in small or large quantities, and turnkey extracting systems can be purchased to simplify the process. It is also possible to make water hash using home-gathered equipment, but with inexpensive kits available, the savings are often negligible. Pre-made systems offer increased precision and efficiency for the water hash process, and their availability contributed to a surge in water hash's popularity during the late 1990s and early 2000s.

Water hash's two decade run of dominance ended with the rise of solvent-extracted hash; shatter, wax, and other butane hash-oils have muscled aside bubble hash on many dispensary shelves in the United States over the last few years. But this competition from solvent hash has also inspired water hash makers to step their game up, inspiring an increased emphasis on appearance and flavor. Ultra-fine water hash is now being sold as "solventless wax," reflecting the broad demand for solvent-free products that mirror the desirable consistency and refined flavor profile of solvent-extracted hash.

High-grade water hash is also great for edibles, and any experienced dabber will tell you that "five star" hash is very dabbable.

It's also next to impossible to seriously injure yourself or anyone else making water hash, because the process doesn't involve any flammable chemicals or potentially explosive machinery.

HOW WATER HASH WORKS

All water hash methods use water, ice, and agitation to separate resin glands from plant material. Water and plant material are placed in a bucket that has been lined with filtration bags, similar in composition to the screens used for making dry sift kief. Like those screens, the bags filter the glands by micron size, separating the hash from the trash. A micron is one-millionth of a meter, or .001 millimeters. The material is stirred to knock the trichomes free, and while the plant material floats in the top bag, the glands (which are heavier) sink and are collected in the lower bags.

Ready-made systems use multiple bags that sort the glands by size: Unlike kief making, the material is separated in one step rather than through repeated sieving. Usually the material is processed once, but some commercial hash makers process it a second time to further isolate the THC.

As with all extraction methods, cold temperature is a key element of water hash production. The ice keeps the water and material very cold so the glands remain brittle and snap off with agitation. After the material is agitated in ice water, it's allowed to settle. Then the bags are separated, and the glands are removed from each one. After the water hash is dried, it's ready to smoke.

Water hash varies in color and can be many shades of white, brown, red, even purple. When extracted from the finest-grade material, the potency of water hash can test as high as many solvent hash products, with up to 80% cannabinoid content.

A NOTE ON YIELDS

Processing 227 grams of high-quality material usually yields between 18 grams (5% yield) to 35 grams (15% yield). Yields increase with the quality of the starting material. However, in some instances, such as with Tangie, obtaining a yield over 7% using water is nearly impossible. This is one reason solvent-based methods and other, newer extraction techniques have overtaken water processing in popularity.

But there are considerations other than yield; the full-spectrum effects and natural flavor profile of water hash are unique because the process preserves the terpenes in the glands. For this reason, some people prefer high-quality water hash to solvent-extracted products.

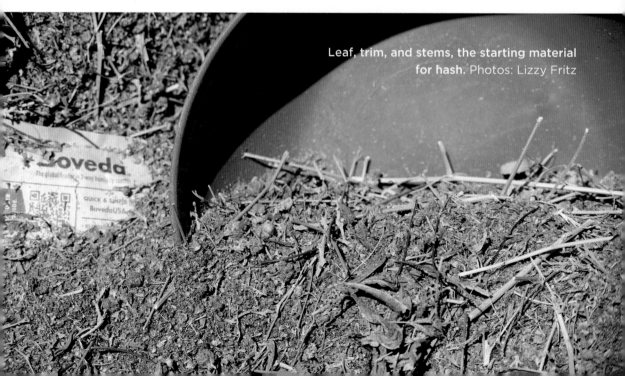

Leaf, trim, and stems, the starting material for hash. Photos: Lizzy Fritz

WATER HASH BASICS

All gland-bearing plant material (leaf, trim, buds, shake, or any combination of the four) can be used to make water hash. Dried or frozen material can also be used.

When making water hash it is important to keep the material and the environment very cold. Heat is the enemy. Low-temperature water, near freezing, makes trichomes brittle enough to snap off. A cool room keeps terpenes from vaping off.

Humidity is also a factor. Avoid humid storage conditions to prevent deterioration from bacteria or molds. One method is to store wet or dried cannabis in the freezer. When using material that has not been stored in this way, place it in the freezer until it gets cold.

It's crucial to treat the cannabis delicately to preserve all of the glands and keep them on the vegetation. Take the utmost care when bucking buds from twigs and stems. Don't mangle the material from excessive trimming or grinding. Coarsely chopped cannabis is most convenient. Remove twigs, stems, and twist ties, because they can tear the hash-making bags.

Whether using a ready-made bag system or materials from your kitchen, the basic principles of making water hash are the same. There are slight contributions by technique, patience, and proficiency, but what primarily determines the quality of the hash you produce is the caliber of the plant material and the quality and size of the filter.

READY-MADE BAGS

For water hash, the ready-made bag systems are an excellent choice. They can be used many times.

Bubble Bags are the design of Fresh Headies in Canada. Bubbleman, the head hash master of Fresh Headies, has traveled extensively, spreading the good word of water hash. He can

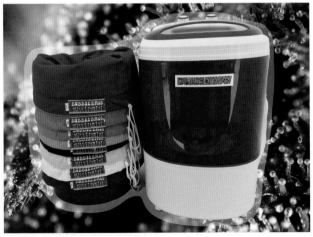

Bubble Bags feature top quality medical grade monofilament screens ranging from 25 to 220 microns. Kits come in your choice of 1, 5, or 20 gallon sizes, with blotting screens.

also be found moderating in online forums on this topic. Bubble Bags are available in one-gallon, five-gallon, and twenty-gallon sizes. All filtration systems are available in sets of four or eight bags and as singles.

There are several other brands of bags. The eight-bag system separates hash into finer categories. The size difference between just-ripe THC glands and overly mature or premature ones allows them to be separated into grades.

USING BUBBLE BAGS

First, the coarse filter bag is secured in a bucket and the water, ice, and plant material are added. The cannabis is agitated using a kitchen mixer or a drill with a paint-mixing attachment — it's worth noting that hash "purists" deplore this level of agitation. After the material settles, the starter bag is pulled out and squeezed. The bulk of the plant material now held in this bag is set aside. This material can be processed again, but the resulting product will be lower grade, though still suitable for cooking.

Line the empty bucket with the additional bags. The finest bag goes in first, so it will be on the bottom. The green water is poured into the bucket, lined with the filtering bags. Pull the bags out one by one and collect the material in the bottom of each one. Allow the end product to dry. Toss the water out or use it for watering plants.

HOME-MADE BAGS

It is possible to make your own bags or to make a smaller amount of water hash without using bags at all. To make bags, acquire silk screen in the appropriate mesh size. Standard silk-screen material is available in several size increments between the desired 100 to 150 strands per inch. The screen must be attached to a tightly woven, water-resistant material (nylon works well) so that the silk screen forms the bottom of the bag. Multiple bags can be made with different screening levels in the 50- to 150-micron range for separating the water hash by quality. The finest screen produces the purest hash. Multiple bags should be designed to fit inside one another, with the finest mesh bag being the largest, and the coarsest mesh bag being the smallest. A separate bag made for coarse filtering (200–250-micron-sized gaps) is used to separate the bulk of the vegetation from the glands in the first phase. This bag should line the bucket. It does not get layered with the other bags, so it should be as large as the bucket allows.

VARIATIONS ON A THEME: OTHER DIY METHODS OF WATER HASH PRODUCTION

Any overview of the water hash-making process would be incomplete without mentioning the many alternate variations on water hash—all of which use slightly different methods to combine water and agitation. Many of these methods sprung from the DIY ingenuity of home hash makers. These methods include the jar shaker method, the coffee filter method, the bucket method, and the blender method.

THE JAR SHAKER METHOD

The simplest method for making water hash is using a homemade shaker. This method is the easiest in terms of time and equipment, but it also produces the least amount of hash, and the product won't be as pure as with methods using micron-gauged filtering bags. Manual agitation is more labor intensive, but it requires no electricity and can be accomplished anywhere that the materials can be gathered.

EQUIPMENT

- Up to an ounce of brittle, dry trim, bud bits, or shake
- Water
- Ice
- Sealable glass jar
- Colander or wire-mesh strainer
- Slotted spoon or tea strainer
- Coffee cone (#4)
- Paper coffee filters
- Dish towel
- Paper towels
- Scraping tool (spoon, credit card, or business card)

METHOD

Grind the marijuana to a coarse powder, similar to dried cooking herbs such as oregano or basil, using a bud grinder, coffee grinder or blender for a very short time.

Place the material in the jar, up to 1 quarter full. Pint, quart, and 2 quart jars all work. Add equal amounts of ice and very cold water until the jar is almost full. Leave about an inch of space at the top of the jar, then seal it and shake for 10 minutes.

Pour the water/material mix into a bowl and put it in the refrigerator to allow it to settle for an hour. Most of the ice may melt in this time.

Remove the floating plant material with a tea strainer or slotted spoon. The plant material can be saved and reprocessed. Manual shaking does not remove all trichomes on the first round.

Once the plant material has been removed, allow the silt to resettle at the bottom of the bowl for 15–20 minutes. Drain off one-half to two-thirds of the water slowly, with an eye to saving all of the silt-like water hash material in the bottom of the jar.

Set up the cone lined with a paper coffee filter. Pour the contents of the bowl through the cone slowly. As the water hash collects in the bottom of the filter, the water will drain more slowly. Allow all of the water to drain from the filter. Then remove the filter from the cone, allowing it to flatten with the wet hash inside. Set it on a dish towel and carefully remove as much water as possible by pressing with the towel or paper towels.

Split the coffee filter along the seam and open it like a butterfly spreads its wings. Collect the material inside using a spoon or card to scrape it loose from the paper. The material is easier to separate from the coffee filter when it's dry or slightly damp.

The material can dry either before or after it's removed from the filter. Even if some of the material is collected for use before the drying completes, the water hash should be allowed to air dry over a day or two to reduce the chance of mold. After the water hash is dry, it can be used, stored, or pressed into hash.

THE COFFEE FILTER METHOD

The coffee filter method works well for small-scale water hash production and uses common kitchen equipment.

Chop the plant material to a coarsely ground consistency. Cone-type coffee makers look like a pointier version of a standard coffee maker basket. They are inexpensive and are available at kitchenware stores, some gourmet coffee shops, grocery stores, or on the web. The #4 size or larger is recommended. Both reusable and disposable filters for these cones are available at the same shops where the cone was purchased.

This method yields nice hash, but not like the product of the precise micron-sized filters of bubble bags. Also, there is no final filtration of small vegetative matter, so the product is not as pure as the hash made in a bag system. Still, water hash produced using this method is equal in quality to dry-screened kief.

EQUIPMENT
- Ice
- Cold water
- Dried plant material (coarsely ground)
- Blender
- Mixing bowl
- Colander or wire-mesh strainer
- Cone-type single-cup coffee maker
- Reusable metal cone coffee filter, or silk screen
- Coffee filters
- 2–3 large glass jars with tight-sealing lids
- Dish towel
- Paper towels
- Scraping tool (spoon, credit card, or business card)

THE BUCKET METHOD

The essentials of water hash methods are the same, whether using a ready-made system or working from your own homemade bags.

EQUIPMENT

- Ice
- Cold water
- Hydrogen peroxide
- 2 buckets with at least one lid
- Dried bud/trim/leaf material
- Handheld mixer or drill with paint-mixing attachment
- Bag system
- Long rubber gloves
- Large towel
- Roll of paper towels
- Spoon or plastic card

METHOD

First, clean and sterilize the buckets and equipment. Mix 10 ounces (1¼ cups) of 3% hydrogen peroxide per quart of water to make a rinse.

If you're using a bag in the first round, place this bag in the bucket. Add equal amounts of ice and water until the bucket is two-thirds full. Add the prepared plant material. Wearing the long rubber gloves, use your hands to submerse it evenly in the ice water. Up to 3½ ounces (100 grams) of plant material can be used in a 5 gallon bucket.

One convenient tool for agitating the mix is a kitchen mixer. Another choice for agitating the water is a drill with paint mixer attachment. A larger mixing tool, powered by an industrial drill is used for the 20 gallon bags. Punch hole(s) in the bucket lid to accommodate the mixing attachments. This keeps the material from sloshing out while it's being agitated and allows the mixer to run hands-free.

Agitate the material for 15 minutes and then allow the mixture to settle. If using a ready-made system, the speed recommended in the instructions should be used. As a general rule of thumb, lower speeds work well when mixing amounts under 5 gallons. Medium to high speeds are better when using a system that is 5 gallons or larger. As it is mixed, the material becomes frothy. You may want to remove the suds before recommencing.

Blend the material up to 4 times for 15 minutes at a time. Mixing the material more times produces higher yields, but also results in more particulate vegetative matter. Longer times produce less pure results, especially if multiple bags aren't separating the hash into grades. With a single collection mechanism, a shorter time should be used on the first round. After this hash is collected, the plant material can be reprocessed using a longer mixing time. Multiple bags allow the material to be processed all at once without sacrificing a high-grade collection.

After the mixing round is completed, let the mixture sit for at least 30 minutes to give the glands time to sink into the collection filters. If most of the ice has melted add more. In cold weather the bucket can be set outside to keep the mixture cold.

Once the material has settled, it's time to separate the glands. If the agitation has been done inside a bag, pull out this bag, removing the bulk of the plant material. The bucket now contains green water with silt in the bottom. This silt is the water hash and a small amount of particulate vegetative matter.

Line the second bucket with the collection bags. The finest mesh bag goes on the bottom, so it's added to the bucket first. The coarsest bag is the last bag added, so it's the top layer. The first bag has separated out everything over the 200–250-micron size, depending on its mesh size. Now the successive layers of the bags will do the grading for you.

Pour the water into the bucket that is lined with the filter bags. Slowly lift out each bag, allowing time for the water to drain. Be patient. If the entire bottom of the bag seems to be clogged it may be necessary to reach in and gently push some material to the side. Stir up the material as little as possible.

After each bag is removed, lay it on the towel and pat off excess water. Wrap it with towels and squeeze it to remove more water. The inside of each bag contains some tan to brown silt-like material. Carefully arrange the bag so that the material is accessible. Blot the material off with a paper towel. Remove it from the bag using a credit card or a spoon. If multiple bags were used, keep the grades separated.

Place the material in a flat-bottomed bowl, or on a plate or other surface where it can be left to dry, then put it in a cool, dark place where it will get some airflow but won't blow away once dry. The material will appear dry in about 12 hours, but allow a full week to completely dry and cure. Allow the moisture to evaporate from the remaining material by keeping it open to air in a cool space to prevent mold growth.

THE BLENDER METHOD

Place enough plant material in the blender to fill it halfway. Add ice and cold water in equal amounts until the blender is full. Turn the blender on at full speed for 45 seconds to a minute. Let the mixture settle. Repeat 3 or 4 times. The more times the blender runs, the higher the yield.

Pour the mixture from the blender through a colander or strainer into a mixing bowl. Bowls designed to pour, such as a pancake batter bowl or a 1–2 quart measuring cup, work best. This step separates out the bulk of the plant material.

Pour the water through the reusable coffee filter into the glass jars until they are about two-thirds full. Sealable glass canning jars work well. Smaller vegetative matter will collect in the coffee filter. However, the glands are small and pass through the reusable coffee filter into the glass jars. After pouring the water/trichome mix through the filter, pour two more cups of water through the filter so remaining trichomes pass through it.

Seal the jars. Place them in the refrigerator for an hour. The glands settle and form silt at the bottoms. Tapping the jars lightly a few times on a tabletop helps settle some of the floating material.

Remove the jars from the refrigerator without stirring up the material that has collected at the bottom. Pour off the top two-thirds of the water. The goal is to retain the glands that are gathered in the bottom while removing as much water content as possible.

Set up the cone on top of a suitable container such as a quart jar. Drain the remaining water and silt through the coffee filter with a disposable filter paper. The flow of water through the filter slows as the material collects; allow it to drain completely.

Carefully remove the paper coffee filter from the cone. Flatten it with the material inside by patting it with a towel.

Material can be dried before or after it's collected from the coffee filter. Drying it inside the coffee filter takes a little longer but the hash is protected from blowing away and is easier to remove from the paper when both are dry. To dry in the coffee filter place it atop a layer of paper or cloth towels. Once it's dry, split the filter along a seam.

Collect the material using a spoon or plastic card. Allow the material to fully dry before pressing or storing, which takes a day or two depending on the environmental conditions and the amount being dried.

WATER HASH DO'S AND DON'TS

- Fresh-frozen material works best. If it was not stored in the freezer, place it inside until it's frozen.
- Use a standard two-beater mixer, a drill with a paint-mixing attachment, or blender.
- Don't get impatient in the final steps! Dry the material thoroughly at the end of the process. Water hash stored before it is dried molds, ruining it.
- Water and mash left over at the end of the process contain nutrients present in the plant material. It's great for watering plants, using as mulch, or adding to compost.

TIPS

Use a siphon rather than a pour to remove one-half to two-thirds of the water from the container. This gives you more control and creates less turbulence so the silt at the container bottom is not disturbed. Use clean, flexible aquarium tubing. Place the other end of the tubing into a sink or other drainage area.

Heat speeds up the drying process. Use a propagation mat, usually used to sprout seedlings—it will maintain a 74°F (23°C) temperature—or a heating pad set on low. Place the mat under a towel and put the drying water hash on top. Food dehydrators set on low are another effective controlled heat source.

INTRODUCTION TO ADVANCED WATER HASH

Water hash produced using advanced methods can definitely hold its own against solvent-extracted hash: In the 2013 Emerald Cup — a longtime, outdoor organic medical marijuana competition in Northern California — the first and second-place water hash winners tested at 67% and 70% THC, a level of potency once thought impossible for old-school water hash.

Advanced water hash uses the same principles outlined in the previous section, it just takes into account more variables, from the strain type and trichome shape to harvest methods and ambient temperature and humidity in the washing room.

THE MACHINE METHOD

There are several key principles for producing the highest-quality, dabbable water hash.

First, trichomes must be treated gently. Mechanical agitation in the ice-bath stage is needed, but it's also the enemy. Paint mixers are too rough for award-winning bubble.

Second, heat is an enemy; it can dry out buds and sap them of their flavors and strength. During drying, high temperatures vaporize hash's great flavors. Storing hash at a high temperature degrades its flavor and potency.

High-grade water hash is being rebranded as "solventless wax," because it gives consumers who want to dab a tasty, effective alternative to BHO and provides producers with a method that doesn't involve flammable solvents or high-pressure machinery.

EQUIPMENT

- 20-gallon Bubble Now, Bubble Magic Extraction Machine, Bubbleator, or top-loading washing machine
- Bubble Bags (microns — 220 zippered to hold the material in the washer; 160, the first filter, removes contaminants; 73 for high grade; 25 for lower grade)
- Cannabis (1,000 to 2,500 grams, frozen, high-trichome leaf)
- Water (filtered for best results)
- Ice—enough to fill the machine 60% full, and refill it as it melts
- 20-gallon bucket
- Alcohol or hydrogen peroxide
- Gloves
- Spoon
- Sieve
- Parchment paper
- Thick cardboard

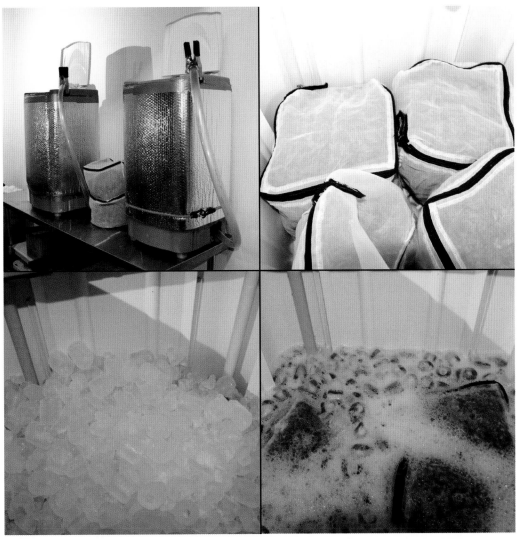

Industrial water hash machines. Mesh bags filled with cannabis inside the machine. Ice filled and then water filled, the bags are ready for agitation. Photos: The Dank Duchess

METHOD

- Consider the best location for setting up the machine. The best situation is a sterile lab setting:
- Hash is very sticky and captures contaminants floating in the air, such as dander, dog hair, and dust, so a room with filtered air is best. The ambient temperature is best below 65°F (18°C) with low humidity—between 15% and 50%. Hash is oxidized and darkens when it's manufactured or stored for long periods at high temperatures such as 80°F to 90°F (27°C to 32°C).
- Next, consider the source material. Dried, cured, sugar leaf works fine, but the

best water hash is made from fresh-frozen material. Trichome-rich leaves are cut from ripe plants, bagged in plastic freezer bags and frozen. Freezing locks in all the terpenes and cannabinoids present on the plant at the time of harvest; significant amounts amounts of both are generally lost to drying, curing, and processing.

- Thoroughly disinfect the machine, hose, bags, and buckets using hydrogen peroxide.
- Line your 20-gallon bucket with filter bags, starting with the finest 25-micron bag and ending with the biggest 160-micron bag.
- Place the machine's outflow hose into the filter bucket.
- Place a base layer of ice in the machine.
- Fit the open, 220-micron bag in the machine and add the material.
- Fill the bag half-full with 9 parts trim to one part ice. Alternate adding trim and ice. Zip up and tie the top of the bag and pour more ice over the bag until the ice level reaches 8 inches below the rim of the machine.
- Add water until it's 4 inches below the surface of the ice. Wait 15 minutes for the trim to soak up the water, then add more ice and water, until the water is below the ice's surface level, and the ice is 8 inches below the rim of the metal basin. Leave room for the mixture to agitate.
- Turn the machine on gentle and monitor the agitation. Use wooden spoons to help the bag settle into the ice bath. Add more ice and water as the ice melts and settles. The color of the water should turn completely gold quickly. On a standard washing machine, use the gentle cycle. DO NOT let the device automatically drain. Run 2 gentle agitation cycles—then let it drain.
- During this ice-cold agitation process, the brittle, frozen trichomes will have snapped off the leaf, traveled through the lining of the 220-micron "garbage" bag, and into the ice bath. The water turns green, and the plant oils make the surface of the water frothy.
- After agitation, the machine pumps the trichome-rich water out of the washer basin and into the filter bags, which are set up inside the 20-gallon bucket.
- The inside of the bucket will be foamy with cannabis oils. Jiggle the bucket gently to help water pass through the filters, and use filtered ice water in a small pump sprayer to rinse the trichomes off the bag's sides and down and through the 160-micron filter.
- Start pulling the bags up one at a time. First pull out the 160-micron bag. The material inside the bottom of the bag looks like grey-green silt. Rinse down the edges, get everything collected in the bottom, and scoop up the resin.
- Pull the second bag, then spray, jiggle, and repeat. The 73–159-micron stuff is a little green, but not as green as the first bag. Keep pulling, spraying, and

jiggling until it's all collected in the middle of the mesh. Trichomes smaller than 70 microns pass through the mesh, but everything from 73 to 159 microns will be collected. This is the sweet spot for trichomes. Solventless competitions are won most frequently by entries collected from the 73, 90, and 120-micron bags. However, narrow-leaf varieties have smaller trichomes, so they tend to have the nicest resin in the range of 25 and 89 microns.

- Pull the bag up. It'll be heavy with water, its pores clogged with trichomes. Slowly spin the emulsion while spraying down the sides. The mesh holds on to the glands while the fine green particles fall through with the water. Keep spraying, rotating, and pulling until the green is gone, leaving what looks like a bunch of golden sand.

- Pull up the bag to the top and spoon out the wet paste onto parchment paper set on a towel or thick cardboard, or something else that will safely wick moisture away.

- The next bag catches the bulk of trichomes between 25 and 73 microns. The material in here is a combination of green contaminant and gold trichomes. The goal is to have the green pass through the screen while retaining the gold. As with the last bag, pull the bag up; it'll be heavy with water. Its pores will be clogged with trichomes. Slowly spin the emulsion while spraying down the sides. The mesh holds on to the glands while the fine green particles fall through with the water. Keep spraying, rotating, and pulling until the green is gone and it looks like a bunch of golden sand.

- Remove this light clay-like wet hash from the mesh and place it on a 25-micron drying screen.

TIPS

- Check the seams to make sure your bubble bags are not inside out.
- Inspect the machine output hose line for leaks.
- Use a gravity-based system with suspended bags and buckets to save your back.
- Buy bags with lots of mesh area, durable sidewalls, and consistent micron spacing—cheap eBay bags often have inconsistent micron widths in the center of the mesh versus the edge.
- Keeps hands off the trichomes.
- Trim wet and freeze.
- If you make water hash often, invest in an ice-making machine.
- You don't have to use as much ice when using large cubes. They don't melt as fast as small pieces.
- **Strains:** Different strains yield differently sized and shaped trichomes, and dif-

fering amounts of oils and terpenes. Hashing Blue Dream versus hashing Bubba Kush is like night and day at the micron level. Blue Dream trichomes are long and thin, and you can raise the temperature and humidity during drying. Bubba Kush, Sour Diesel, and OG Kush glands are short, stocky, and oily, and need to be processed at as cold a temperature as possible and dried at 40°F (4°C) under minimal humidity to capture the resin's odors.

- **Bag Size and Number:** This can vary. You can use as few as 225 and 160-micron bags, plus a 220-micron garbage bag for simplicity's sake, or pull and spoon progressively narrower bands of glands and materials at 190, 120, 90, 73, and 45 microns.

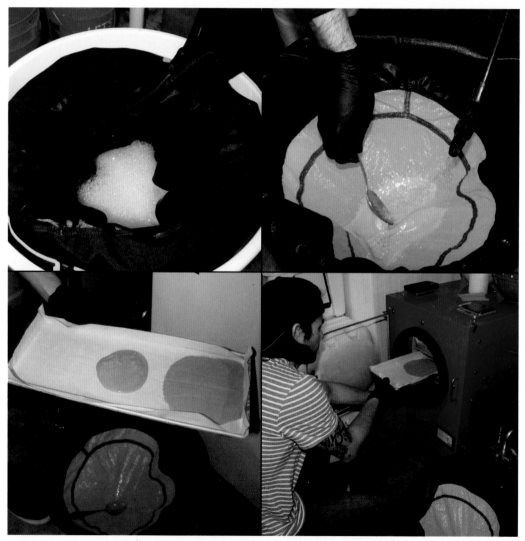

Cold water is added to rinse away bubbles from agitation and then a finer spray to collect the glands at the bottom of the bag. Water hash is scooped out of the bag for drying. Placing hash into the freezer to finish drying. Photos: The Dank Duchess

- **Agitation:** Purists sometimes use something as basic as a pole or paddle to gently hand-agitate the main bag in the bucket; the trade-off is in the yield. A 30-minute machine wash of 1,000 high-quality grams can yield as much as 112 grams of top-shelf hash. Less agitation equals purer hash but lower yield.

DRYING

There's a compromise in drying. Trying to remove moisture from the hash without vaporizing the delicious yet volatile essential oils, or terpenes.

Drying should be done in a room with a temperature between 40°F (4°C) and 68°F (20°C). The reason for the low temperature is that some terpenes evaporate at 70°F (21°C).

Humidity is also a factor, with 30-45% humidity being optimal, but it can vary by strain.

Drying effectively is accomplished in a number of ways, including the chop, sieve, microplane, and freeze drying methods.

ADVANCED METHODS OF DRYING

CHOP METHOD

The chop method is accomplished by chopping damp resin into small pieces so that it can be spread over a wide surface area.

In a cold room, using a small knife, chop the resin swiftly, creating rows of damp material. Then shape rows perpendicular to the first row. On a swatch of parchment paper, spread the chopped resin over the surface, taking care to keep the clumps as separate as possible. If a wide surface area is not available, resin can be dried in pizza boxes. Cardboard boxes wick away moisture well and are effective for protecting drying resin from light and contaminants. The chop method is the least effective method for thoroughly drying the resin because clumps tend to trap moisture.

SIEVE METHOD

Using the sieve method results in very small clumps of resin that do dry thoroughly.

Place 2 strainers and 3 spoons in the freezer. After the wash, resin has been drying on the 25 micron screen. Wrap the screen around the resin and wrap again in a clean paper towel. Place it in the refrigerator for 2 hours. To utilize the sieve method, the material has to be cold and devoid of excess moisture.

After 2 hours, take one of the frozen strainers and spoons out of the freezer, and the resin out of the refrigerator. Place the partially dried resin in one of the strainers. Using a circular motion, lightly run the cold spoon over the mass of resin. A fine rain of resin will fall onto the parchment paper (or pizza box).

Sour Banana Hash, 70-micron screen. Photo: Nikka T

Continue to cover the parchment in a light dusting of resin powder, taking care not to pile resin on top of itself. When the resin begins either sticking to the strainer or the spoon, exchange for a fresh, frozen instrument. When resin warms, it sticks together, making sieving nearly impossible, so work quickly.

Allow resin to dry between 3 and 14 days, depending on the strain and the conditions of the room. When resin is dry, it sounds like sugar crystals when poured.

ZESTING (MICROPLANE) METHOD

A favorite among many hash makers, the zesting method consistently allows the resin to dry thoroughly.

Place three lemon zesters and the resin that has been resting on the drying screen in the freezer. It's important that the puck be frozen. The next day, in a cold room, remove a zester and a puck. Using quick movements, grate the resin over a large swath of parchment paper (or pizza box).

Allow resin to dry between three and 14 days, depending on the strain and the conditions of the room. When resin is dry, it sounds like sugar crystals when poured.

The main drawback of the microplane method is that the trichome heads are sliced open, thereby allowing terpenes to escape. Also, ripped heads are less stable, leading to shortened shelf life.

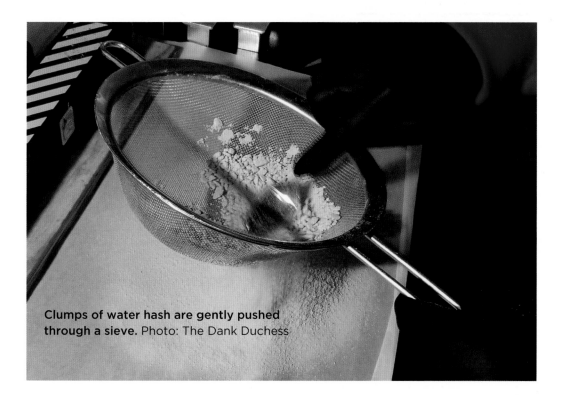

Clumps of water hash are gently pushed through a sieve. Photo: The Dank Duchess

FREEZE-DRYING METHOD

Freeze drying has only recently become a viable option for getting resin to its absolute driest. The basic idea behind freeze drying is to have water frozen inside resin pucks sublimate to vapor, completely bypassing the liquid stage. Over the course of about 24 hours frozen resin becomes like dry sand.

With whichever process used, the key is to achieve complete drying. Under magnification, the final product will look like sandy heaps of full, sticky, oily, trichome heads. Store in a cool, dark place, and don't press until the material is completely dry.

PRESSING AND STORAGE—THE FINAL STEP

Concentrated cannabis is the future of cannabis. As covered above, water and ice can be used to mechanically separate trichomes from the plant, and filters can concentrate the glands into unpressed or "loose" hash. Further refinement using machinery and tighter control of temperature and humidity will yield the strongest nonsolvent concentrates. Pressing unrefined hash into balls, cakes, or slabs creates hashish; all steps of the process are consumable, but making hashish is a two-step process: First, the glands are collected; second, the collected material is compressed into into bricks or balls.

Pressing hash involves a combination of force and mild heat to condense the glands into a solid mass. The shape and size of hash varies depending on the pressing method. When hand pressed, hash is often ball-shaped. Flat-pressed hash may look like thin shale rock, with hardened shelf-like layers that chip along the creases. Mechanically pressed hash is usually a neat cake, like a bar of soap.

Hashish ranges in color and pliability. The variety of marijuana used, manufacturing method, temperature, and the purity of the kief influence its color, which ranges from light yellow-tan to charcoal black, and its texture, which ranges from pliable taffy to hard and brittle.

Hashish oxidizes and darkens from exposure to light, oxygen, and heat. Regardless of its texture, high-quality hash should soften with the simple warmth of your hands.

Aficionados often describe the high that hash produces as more complex than that of kief. In the region of traditional hash making kief is typically aged, sometimes for a year or more, before it's pressed. Most modern hash makers do not wait that long.

TIP

Unpressed kief oxidizes in warm temperatures, while hash is more resilient to warmth, so long as it's pressed when it's totally dry. When pressed wet, however, hash molds. You can store material in its unpressed form in a cool, dark place. Once pressed, hash stored in the freezer suffers little from aging.

PREPARING KIEF OR WATER HASH FOR HASH MAKING

Before attempting to press kief or water hash the material must be completely dry. To ensure that all moisture has been eliminated before pressing, dry the material one last time. Place the kief or water hash in a food dehydrator set on the lowest setting, or a horticultural heat mat (preset at 74°F [23°C]), microwave the material on low, or place it in an open dish in a frost-free freezer. The vacuum conditions promote water evaporation, preventing mold from infecting and spoiling the hash. However, when the drying temperature is above 75°F (24°C), some of the terpenes will evaporate, diminishing the kief's unique odors and their effects.

Pressing transforms the material both chemically and physically; the glands are warmed and most break, releasing the sticky oils that contain the psychoactive cannabinoids, as well as the terpenes—the source of cannabis's smell, taste, and suite of effects.

Terpenes lend fragrance to the hash. Smells and flavors characteristic to hashish range from spicy or peppery to floral. Many terpenes are volatile at room temperature. When inhaled, they contribute to the lung expansiveness (cough factor), as well as the taste. Aged kief is both milder in smell and flavor, and less cough inducing, because some of the terpenes (but not the THC) have dissipated.

Releasing and warming cannabinoids exposes them to air. This has the beneficial effect of potentiating the THC through decarboxylation. Continued exposure to light, air, heat, and moisture leads to THC deterioration.

You can press hash manually or mechanically. Manual methods work well for smaller amounts. Mechanical methods use a press, which is fast, convenient, and efficient. This section describes a reliable manual method and covers mechanical pressing.

SHOE HASH METHOD

This pressing method lets you multitask. While you're busy doing other things, the hash is being inconspicuously pressed within your shoe!

Shoe hash is a low-hassle way to press a small amount of kief or water hash. A few grams, usually 5 grams or less, are bagged in tightly wrapped cellophane or parchment paper wrapped around the material several times. A piece of tape stops it from unfolding. Punch a pinhole through the package to allow trapped air to escape. Don't use a plastic bag because the hash sticks to it messily. It's important for scientific as well as psychological reasons for the material to be securely sealed before it goes in your shoe.

Place the package inside the heel of your shoe. Hard-soled shoes or boots are better for pressing than soft-soled shoes, such as sports shoes, which take longer to process the kief.

The heel's weight and pressure within the shoe, aided by body heat, presses the hash into a slab. The pressing takes 15 minutes to an hour of on-foot activity, but it benefits from additional wear.

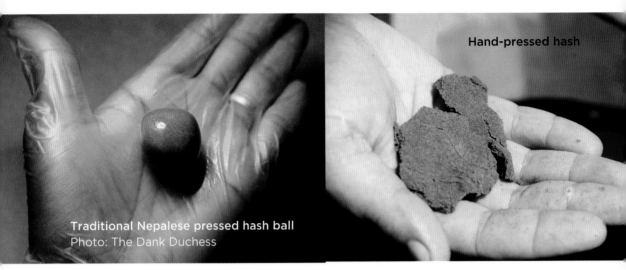

Hand-pressed hash

Traditional Nepalese pressed hash ball
Photo: The Dank Duchess

PRESSING BY HAND METHOD

Pressing by hand is a method for transforming kief into hashish a few grams at a time. Pressing by hand is convenient since it requires no additional equipment but it takes considerable energy and the results are better with a practiced technique. Those unaccustomed to hand pressing may find it difficult to make the material bind together. The considerable work it takes to get well-pressed hash can easily result in sore hands.

This method works best using freshly sieved medium to high-quality kief. If the kief contains a significant amount of vegetative material, it's harder to mold into hash and may not stick together properly. To hand press, measure out a small mound of fresh kief that will fit comfortably in the hand, usually a few grams at the most. Work this material with one hand against the other until it begins to cohere into a solid piece. Then rub it between the palms, or between palm and thumb. After 10 minutes or more of working the material, it begins to change density. Dry, aged kief lacks some of its original stickiness and may take longer to stick together, but if it was stored properly, it should cooperate, though it may require more kneading. When a piece of hashish has not been pressed properly, it crumbles easily at room temperature.

If the kief is particularly stubborn and won't stick together to form a mass, mildly heat it. Wrap the material in food-grade cellophane, ensuring that it is completely sealed and all the air is squeezed out. Wrap this package in several layers of thoroughly wetted newspaper, cloth or paper towels. Turning frequently, warm in a skillet that is set on the lowest heat. It doesn't need to be heated as long as other methods because the only point of heating is to get the material to stick together so it can be kneaded into a solid piece.

Another method is to wrap it the same way and press it for a few seconds on each side with an iron that is set on a very low heat setting.

HOT WATER BOTTLE METHOD

The concept of using the hot water bottle method is similar to pressing by hand. However, more heat is applied to thoroughly melt the waxy cuticle of each trichome head. This method works with medium- to high-quality resin that is bone dry.

Place a pile of resin on the surface of either organic cellophane or parchment paper. Fold the paper in half. Bring water to a boil. Fill a wine bottle with the hot water. Allow the bottle to cool for 5 minutes. Place the hot wine bottle on the paper-covered resin and allow it to sit for 30 seconds.

Look through the bottle to the darkening stain of the warming resin. If the color is changing quickly, you have the sign that the resin will press very quickly. If the resin barely begins to change after 30 seconds, you will have to work the resin considerably more. Using a series of passes, roll the wine bottle over the resin using minimal pressure. Allow the heat to melt the material without forcing, using the pressure of your hand. Flip the paper over and do the same process in the other side.

By now, the resin should no longer be a mound, but flatter and more of a patty: If not completely so. With a swift flip of the wrist, open the paper. The resin should be sticky and have a nice sheen. Fold the resin in half and then again and begin to press once more. Repeat this process one more time before taking the warm resin into the palm of your hand.

To create a modern-day "temple ball," roll the ball like a mass of clay. Roll it with firm pressure; compressing the resin together and pushing out any excess air. Resin that has lumps, lines and wrinkles need to be more thoroughly worked. Continue rolling the resin until you're satisfied with the mass in your hand.

With very high-quality resin, the result will be a completely melted, shiny mass of resin ready for storage.

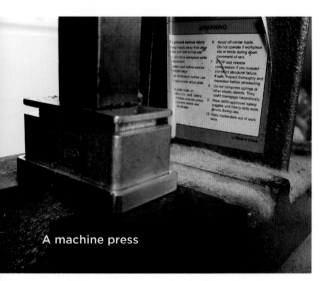

A machine press

MACHINE-PRESS METHOD

Making hash is a cinch with a mechanical press. Bookbinding presses, called nipping presses, can be used. Plans are available on the web for building a press using a hydraulic jack.

Hand-pumped hydraulic presses are a less expensive way to get a tight press. Another cost-effective method uses a vice grip, although it takes some adaptation.

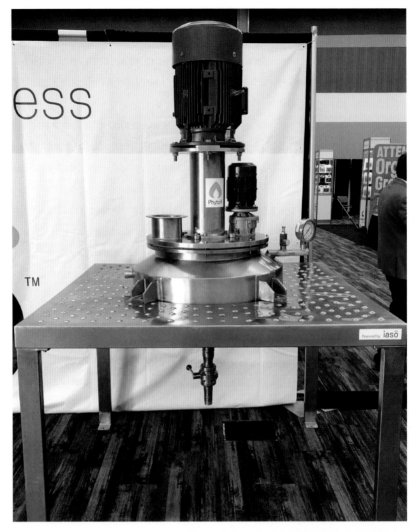

To make concentrates with PhytoX by iASO, cannabis cell fragmentation occurs by intense hydrodynamic force. Hydrodynamic force is a controllable and fast method of extraction that allows more complete penetration into plant tissue. Water can enter the cell transporting essential oils and bio-active compounds producing full spectrum high-potency extracts with the highest contents of phenols, flavonoids, non-flavonoids, carotenoids, terpenoids, phytosterols. Works with fresh or dry plant materials and can process five batches of fifty five pounds a day.

For small amounts, a pollen press can be used in conjunction with a handheld kief-collecting grinder. Kief is added to this small metal tube. The tension pin is placed in, and the pollen press is screwed shut. The next day, the kief has been pressed into a neat hash block. Many companies have similar presses now, including one made of stainless steel with a low-torque T-handle.

STORAGE

Once the hashish is pressed, it can be kept for months or possibly years with little deterioration to its potency and flavor, with proper storage. A frost-free freezer is the best place for storing hash.

Metal, glass, or silicone containers are preferred for storage. Plastics and rubber are not recommended because the terpenes—responsible for the flavor and aroma of the hash—are somewhat volatile compounds that interact chemically with plastic or rubber, degrading both the hash and the container. However, this happens slowly under freezing conditions.

Over time, the outer layer of hashish oxidizes and loses potency. The inside, not exposed to higher levels of light and oxygen, remains potent. Remember that mild light, heat, moisture, and oxygen oxidizes the outside of the hash, destroying its potency.

Making hash is a wonderful method of preserving resin long after cannabis has been harvested. Whether in the kitchen or in the lab, hash making is a process that is available to everyone. Using old school methods or new school techniques, the process is relatively straightforward — agitate to remove trichomes, collect the resin, sort the resin by size, dry the resin, smoke and enjoy!

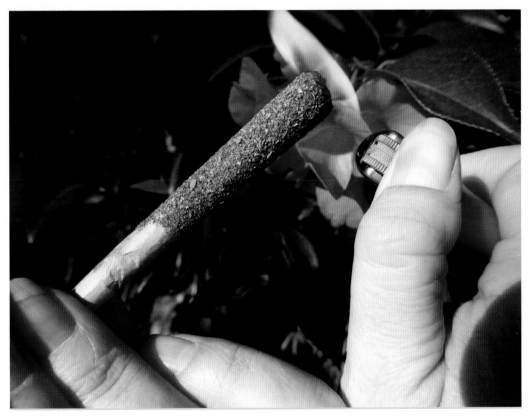

Covered in freshly ground flower, Churros from Your Highness are dipped in solvent-free Gold Drop oil. They pack a punch with a great tasting terpene pairing.

The Original Resinator

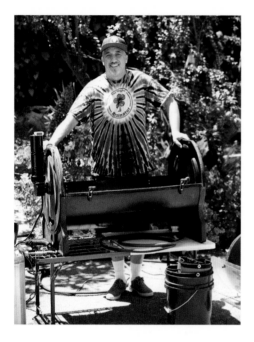

Like so many cannabis-related technologies, the origins of the Resinator was a labor of love. The prototype machine was built in 2008 by Travis Arnovick and James Watts. This original bucket-based contraption was held together by duct tape, bungee cords, silk screen, and paper clips. After they strapped on the engine — an old BBQ rotisserie motor — it was ready to roll. This magnificent beast went through a long series of trials and test runs until the first market-ready Resinator was built in 2011.

Before their Resinator endeavor, the company founders used to spend long days and nights trying to maximize the amount of resin they could extract from trim and shake, and quickly came to the conclusion that there had to be a better way.

"We would go about collecting the resin glands through a variety of old school traditional methods, but these procedures were too labor intensive and time consuming," says Arnovick. "So we thought that there had to be a better way, and wanted to take the manual element out of the equation and make the process mostly mechanical. So we set out to create a solution to this problem."

Today's Resinator is a multi-use, wet/dry, flash freeze, all-in-one, patented, rotary separation apparatus. The machine uses a dry sieve tumble method — aided by ice and water — to extract the essence of botanical resin glands from wet or dried flowers and plant clippings.

The company's uniquely crafted Resin Collection Bags and removable/washable drum screens sift undesired plant material, stems, and particulates, leaving only the desired trichomes to fall through the high-quality, micron-rated monofilament screens. The combination of these methods and ingredients significantly increases yields and efficiency compared to other sifting techniques.

Some of the design features that set the Resinator apart from the competition include its removable/replaceable and washable screens that come in 8 different sizes, depending on the type of extraction or separation that is desired. Another important aspect of the design is the use of liquid CO_2, which allows producers to work with live plant material and extract live resin from uncured biomass. This method of extraction is popular with a variety of rosin techniques, including closed-loop systems, short-path/fractional distillations and ice-wax extractions. The liquid CO_2 allows the machine to instantly freeze, fracture, and extract resin glands and trichomes from cured and uncured plant material, achieving 20% (or better) returns in as little as 10 minutes.

Manufacturers of tinctures, oils, salves, topicals, edibles, and concentrates always prefer pure extracts, and the Resinator delivers high-quality resin all day long. The Resinator can also be employed as a wet/dry flower trimmer, using a mesh screen and CO2 to accomplish up to 85% of the job, while trimming 1 pound per minute.

"We spent countless hours in the field with R&D and went through so many concepts, mold changes, screen designs, and motors," said Arnovick. "Success and failures alike, we stayed diligent in our pursuit of perfection until we finally found the winning combination. We weren't NASA scientists, just a couple of dreamers with passion to bring our ideas to reality."

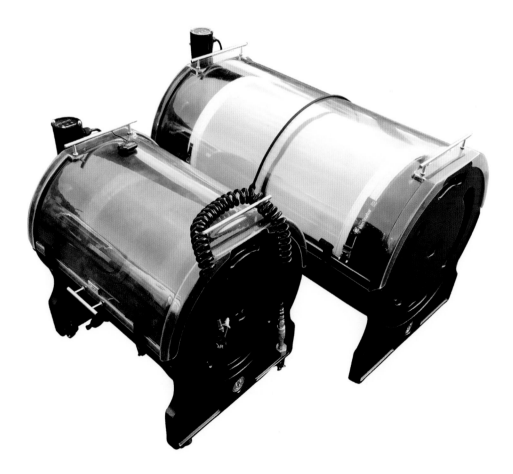

HOW TO USE THE ORIGINAL RESINATOR XL MODEL:

In addition to collecting kief and trimming flowers, The Original Resinator also makes water hash. By adding ice and water you can make bubble hash.

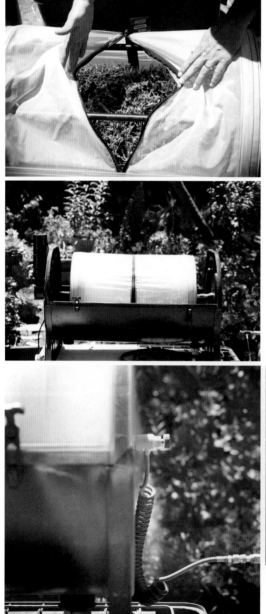

1. Weigh and measure your materials in preparation for water extraction
2. Empty material directly into center chamber of the Resinator and zip up the mesh bag
3. Install the CO_2 coil and make sure to have the temperature diode located somewhere in the chamber
4. Turn the Resinator on to a low speed and inject liquid CO_2 for 30 to 60 seconds
5. It needs to tumble for about a minute per pound of material

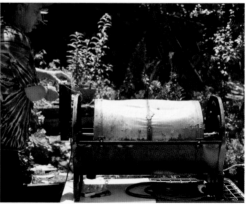

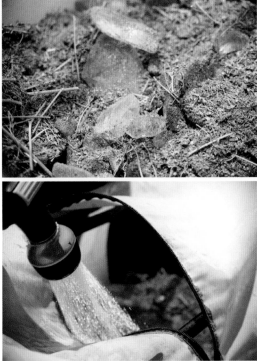

6. After CO_2 injection, add ice and water directly to the chamber and let it tumble for about 20 minutes

7. Take your resin collection bags and put them in a bucket, attach the hose to the Resinator

8. Let the water drain from the chamber into the bags

9. Plug the hose-hole again and repeat the ice and water steps for a second run, let it run for another 5-10 minutes

10. Shake the rest of the water from the bags into the bucket and empty the bags of material onto a tray and let it dry

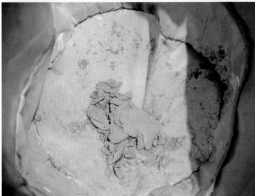

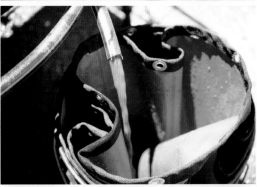

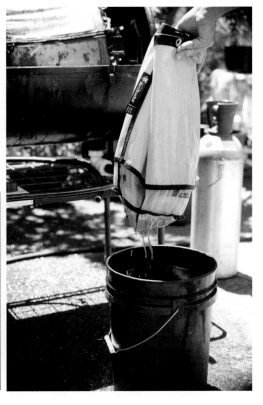

Rosin dripping during a press with Sasquash.
Photo: Fred Morledge

CHAPTER 8

Rosin

Rosin is a concentrated blend of terpenes and cannabinoids extracted using a method sometimes called "rosin tech." It's the simplest, least expensive way to extract concentrate from raw buds or hash for more effective dabbing. Instead of a chemical process, rosin tech relies on heat and pressure to squeeze cannabinoids and terpenes from the source material. It is a very fast process: A batch of rosin can be produced in moments and consumed immediately. Another advantage of rosin production is that it poses minimal risk of physical injury.

The physical science of rosin is simple: Applying heat melts the terpenes and cannabinoids into a pliable resin. Then it is squeezed using a press. Some lipids and waxes melt at the same temperatures. Thus the finished product is generally not as refined as the results of some other methods. One trade-off is the speed and ease of extraction.

There is a wide range of tools and equipment that can be used to make rosin. The choice depends mostly on the quantity being pressed. On the hobby level you can use household items. Industrial processors use pneumatic or hydraulic presses.

No matter the size of the project, the start-up costs of this method are very low compared to chemical extraction, where just the cost of the safety equipment and laboratory modifications exceeds the cost of even an elaborate large-scale rosin operation. However, the costs for the processes of running a solvent extraction setup are lower and the yields higher.

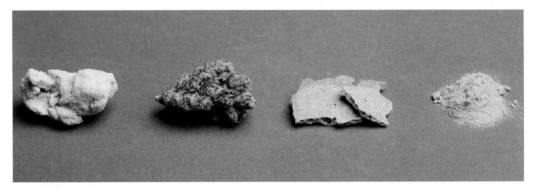

Starting materials used for rosin making. Hash, bud, pressed hash, and kief.
Photo: Fred Morledge

A WORD ON MATERIAL SELECTION AND ROSIN CONSUMPTION SAFETY

A few chapters back we noted that butane extraction is dangerous but BHO is not. Rosin is the inverse because you must be careful about screening material for mold, residual pesticides, and other contaminants. They stick with the resin so they become concentrated in the process. This can cause serious repercussions for the end product and, more importantly, the end *user*.

One feature of hydrocarbon extraction is its ability to strip away or neutralize biological impurities including bacteria, mold, and other contaminants. Moldy but potent trim processed with butane results in a safe product. However, when processed for rosin, there is a buildup of dangerous microbials. Even if you're growing your own starting material, it should be tested for you to know exactly what is present in the rosin.

Many people choose to consume rosin over solvent-extracted products because of perceived health concerns. Some of them do this because of an immunodeficiency or some other medical condition, while others are caught up in a cloud of alarmist "reefer madness" surrounding solvent extraction.

Bottom line: It's crucial that you ensure clean, high-quality source material, whether you're pressing rosin from trim, buds, or hash.

ROSIN 101: THE FLAT IRON TECHNIQUE

The easiest way to understand rosin is to make a small batch on your own. It's simple and requires very little equipment. Let's begin by pressing out some flower rosin — here's what you'll need to get started:

EQUIPMENT FOR BASIC FLOWER ROSIN PRESS:

- **Buds** — for our purposes, use 1-7. Our goal is to learn the process and taste your first homemade product.
- **Tong-style hair-staightener / flat iron** — there are several factors to

consider here, but the biggest obstacles are heat and durability. Some popular models like the Remington have minimum settings too hot to leave the device on during pressing, meaning that you have to warm it, turn it off, and use a laser thermometer "heat gun" to ensure ideal temp. This tool is inexpensive and fun to use. If you don't have access to a heat gun, something inexpensive like the 2-inch model from Conair will allow you to "set and forget" the heat, because the lowest setting is generally cool enough for rosin extraction. However, part of the lower cost comes from a more brittle plastic housing for the heating plates, meaning that the Conair is more susceptible to physical cracking and breakage. A model with a digital temperature readout is also a good choice for irons that do have temp settings low enough for rosin.

- **Parchment paper** — but NEVER wax paper, because you don't want wax to melt into your final product. This will happen if you use wax instead of parchment paper. You can also use silicone mats and other heat-resistant material, but for your first press, parchment is fine.
- **Bar clamp (optional)** — pressure is half of the magic behind rosin, so you have to ensure that you have enough. When pressing small quantities, manual pressure is generally adequate, but for a more efficient press and a higher yield, clamps can be applied to the outside of the iron.
- **Micromesh/silkscreen filters (optional**) — pressing rosin tends to spread the extracted concentrate outward from the buds being pressed, meaning that screens aren't always strictly necessary to keep plant material out of the final product. However, to ensure a product free of particulates, you can wrap your bud in silkscreen or micromesh material. Some people also use unbleached tea bags for these smaller batches of flower rosin.
- **Collection tool** — this can be anything with a flat edge and a roughly nonstick (or easily heatable) surface, so a razor blade or other scraper works well.
- **Protective work gloves** — It's pretty difficult to injure yourself making rosin, especially using this method, but it's not impossible. Wearing work gloves protects your hands from painful burns, which a hair straightener is more than capable of inflicting.

PRESSING FLOWER ROSIN

Plug in the flat iron and set it to the target temperature. If you've selected the basic 2-inch Conair model, set it to "1." If you have a model with a digital temperature display, set it between 280 and 330°F. Check model.

Place your bud inside the tea bag or filter (if applicable), and fold it inside folded parchment paper.

Ensure the iron is still at the appropriate temperature and that the bud is secured in its envelope, then clamp the envelope with the flat iron, focusing the pressure on the buds in the middle. If you're using clamps, tighten them for 3-8 seconds — you'll know you're done when you hear the sizzle sound of resin escaping and interacting with the heat.

Unclamp the iron, open the envelope, and pluck the buds out — this step is another reason many people use bags and filters, because it reduces the opportunity to contaminate an otherwise clean rosin batch while removing plant material.

Take the envelope of warm rosin, refold it, and roll or spread out your rosin as desired. Then place the envelope on a cool surface for a minute or so before opening and collecting the rosin.

Now it's time to dab the rosin! If you have any left when you're done dabbing, keep it in a cool, dark place inside a nonstick container. The main drawback to rosin is that it's best consumed fresh and it doesn't retain its terpenes as well as other cannabis concentrates, so it goes stale quicker, especially when it isn't kept in a cool environment. This is something to consider when deciding how much rosin to make at a time.

THE ROSIN REVOLUTION

Rosin has blossomed in popularity over the last few years because you can quickly make tasty, potent extracts using inexpensive equipment. With training and experience, the product can rival solvent extracts in potency and flavor.

Rosin processing, though not a cold process, occurs below the volatilization point for *most* of the terpenes, and doesn't reach the temperatures needed for decarboxylation, so the rosin is mostly a concentration of THCa and/or CBDa, the acidic precursors to the cannabinoids. The result: the material will not be intoxicating if eaten.

Rosin can also be used to infuse edibles if preparation involves a high enough temperature to decarboxylate the acids. For an edible that doesn't require a hot enough temperature for decarboxylation), predecarboxylate it in the butter or oil being used in the recipe. Place the rosin and the oil or butter on simmer for 15 to 20 minutes to activate the cannabinoids.

STARTING MATERIAL

There are three basic types of material you can press rosin from: buds, hash and kief. Within those categories there are different types and grades.

BUDS

The higher the cannabinoid content of your starting material, the higher yields you can expect. For the best rosin, press the best buds. Small buds and trim can also be pressed into rosin.

Freshly cured, resin-rich material results in the best rosin. It is rich in terpenes and high in cannabinoids. Conversely, older, drier material results in lower yields of a darker, less flavorful rosin that has a different effect than fresh rosin. It is more laid-back, contemplative to sedative. As the starting material aged, most of the cannabinoids decarboxylated. As a result, you can get high from ingesting this rosin without heating it.

HASH

When rosin is pressed from hash, it's a secondary concentration, a refinement of a concentrated product. This results in a higher concentration of cannabinoids in the resulting rosin. For instance, pressing bubble hash often results in shatter-like clarity and terpene profiles. Creating a stunning product requires exceptional starting material; fresh, with a high ratio of oil to plant matter. Never press wet or moist material.

Rosin pressed from water hash collected from different grade filters results in rosins with distinctly different effects.

KIEF

As with hash, kief or sift comes in many quality grades, and as with all starting material, the potency of the product determines the ceiling of yield. Dry sift generally contains a relatively high percentage of plant material. The more plant matter removed from the trichome heads, the higher the yields and the cleaner and smoother the resulting rosin.

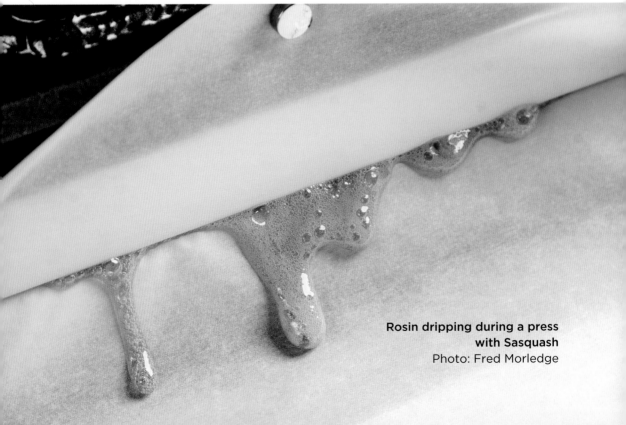

**Rosin dripping during a press
with Sasquash**
Photo: Fred Morledge

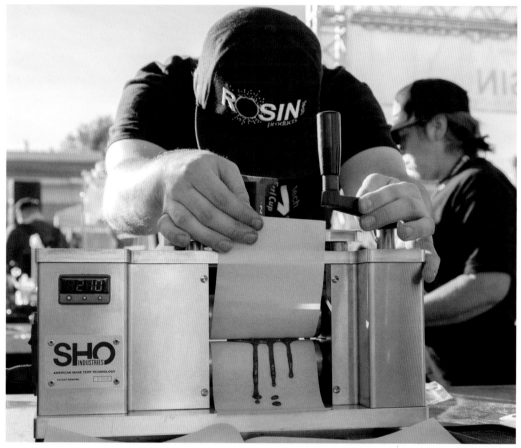

Breaking from the traditional rosin press design, the Rosin Roller uses two heated rollers, reducing the pressure required and allowing for the increased production speed. reducing the need for pressure.

ROSIN 201: MACHINE PRESSING

There are practical limits on how large you can scale up rosin production, but an industrial press that can apply low enough heat and high enough pressure at the same time can be used to press rosin, so those limits correspond with the physical dimensions and specifications of the press.

CHOOSING A PRESS

The first step to picking a rosin press is figuring out how much rosin you're trying to press. Are you making this for personal use, or are you a commercial extractor? Do you plan to press buds, hash, or both?

Don't forget the old hair-straightener technique; even if you're looking to process larger amounts for personal use, most people find they can make more than they need for their head stash using the most basic technology.

If you do choose to purchase a press, a big factor is the amount of pressure it produces. You shouldn't spend money on fancy equipment you don't actually need — you don't buy a

rocket ship to drive to the grocery store, and you shouldn't buy a press that puts out 25 tons of pressure when all you need is 2 to 5 tons, which is all you'll need if you're planning to press hash or small quantities of bud. If you want to press multiple ounces of bud and hash, you'll need more pressure — 10 to 25 metric tons.

Most commercially available rosin-specific presses have been designed to press hash only; if you plan to press flower, make sure you have enough pressure for the amount you plan to press.

While the physical science behind rosin tech is always the same, whether you're using a hair straightener or a 12-ton hydraulic "H-frame" press, the larger scale does necessitate the use of some additional equipment.

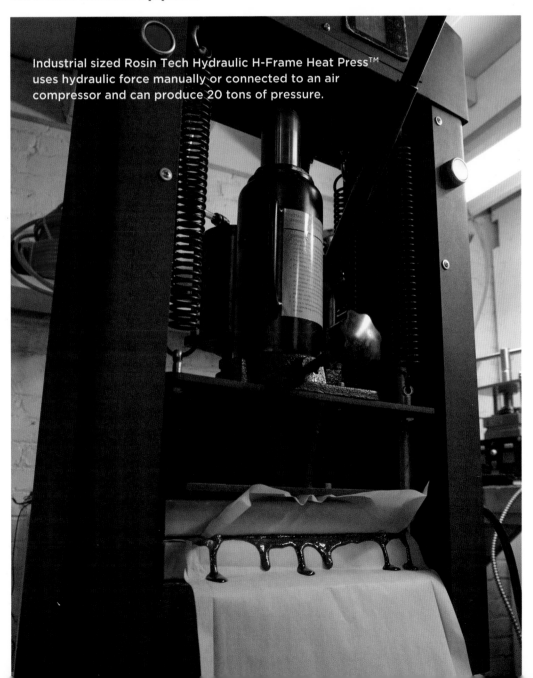

Industrial sized Rosin Tech Hydraulic H-Frame Heat Press™ uses hydraulic force manually or connected to an air compressor and can produce 20 tons of pressure.

Sasquash

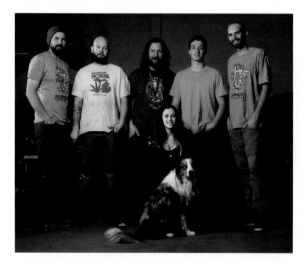

In early 2013, a new and potent type of hash came out. It melted like butter, left nary a trace of residue, and had a golden color and rich taste that created an immediate buzz; "Hash Rosin" was becoming popular. Fast forward to 2015, when Phil Salazar starting pressing flowers; instead of hash, flower rosin was born. Phil Salazar, the creator of flower rosin, knew he had something great. Only occasionally popping up in stores and cannabis events, Phils flower rosin was quickly snapped up, and became a myth within the community. One day Phil and his business partners were brainstorming a name for their new company, which was building one of the first industrial-strength presses to produce flower rosin. "Sasquash" seemed to fit the bill.

Whereas the first wave of oil manufacturers used solvents — most often hydrocarbons (e.g, butane) and CO_2 — to produce full-melt extracts, Salazar took a different route. Striving for a more organic, solventless approach, he started experimenting with a T-shirt press with heated plates to extract the delicate essential oils from cannabis flowers and bubble hash. After multiple successful runs, his cousins Matt and Mike Ilich and Joel Thurman started fabricating commercial machine prototypes at their barn-based production facility in Anza, California. They teamed up with Phil and soon enough, the Sasquash rosin press was born.

In 2016, the team attended their first Cannabis Cup and sold 20 of the machines, and by 2017 the newly formed company, Support the Roots, took home the High Times STASH Award for the best rosin press.

The Sasquash press allows the user to have full control of the temperature and pressure applied to flowers, dry sift, or bubble hash to achieve the highest quality rosin. One of the great benefits of this process is that, you aren't using solvents and can make hash almost instantly. It also preserves the delicate terpenes in the flowers, which makes for a more flavorful and aromatic experience that cannabis connoisseurs pay top dollar for.

From a safety and ease-of-use standpoint, the Sasquash press is certainly one of the best methods for rosin extraction, and it comes in four different sizes — 5 ton, 10 ton, 15 ton, and 25 ton — for producers big and small. Using two heated platens that are compressed at 0 to 25 tons of pressure, the machines can squish 1 gram to 4 ounces at a time. The operator can slowly apply heat and pressure to hash or flowers, and melt the oil into a viscous state through a 35-micron grade nylon screen to produce a golden flow of rosin.

And while most hash-making techniques are too expensive or cumbersome for the DIY crowd, the company markets its products at a price point that makes them attractive for small commercial rosin producers, and even crafty enthusiasts. Indeed, the company's founders had this in mind as they were designing the press.

"We wanted to provide a machine that could make everyone's rosin extracting process easier, along with changing the way people think about the products they're consuming," says Matt Ilich.

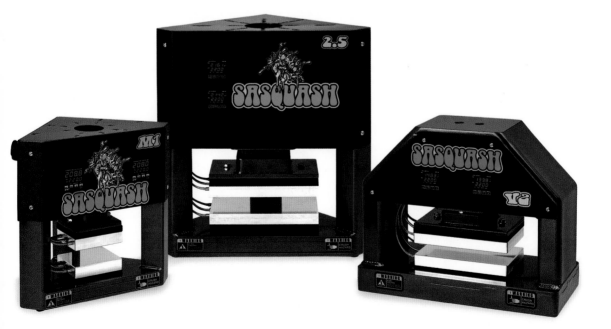

TOOLS FOR MACHINE ROSIN

PRE-PRESS MOLDS

Pre-press molds are a crucial component of many smaller rosin presses. Pressure affects yield, so you want to maximize that pressure by compacting your material into as small and dense a surface area as possible. The smaller you can get it, the more pressure will be exerted during your press.

Think about it this way: You have 14 grams of bud and a press that can exert a metric ton of pressure, 2,000 pounds. If you spread out your 14 grams of material within a 4×4 inch square, it is an area of 16 inches. Divide 16 into 2,000 to determine the surface pressure being exerted on the product by the press, and you get 125 pounds per square inch.

If the 14 grams of material were confined it to a 2×2 in square, an area of four square inches, and pressed with the 2,000 pound press, it is now exerting quadruple the pressure — 500 pounds per square inch.

FILTER BAGS

It's possible to do a "naked press" on a bud—pressing it without any physical screen or filtration to remove plant material. But if you want to further refine your product and confine your material to a condensed area (without the trichome loss incurred using pre-press molds or hand pressing), filter bags are an excellent option and should be used for large quantities that are used in machine presses. They are available in several micron sizes, which like bubble bags used in cold-water extraction, physically isolate a refined slice of the cannabinoids present in the product.

A WORD ON "NAKED PRESSING"

Pressing bud "naked," without a bag, is a bit faster, but very messy and harder to clean up. When pressing naked, you won't do a preheat; allow the platens to meet and give the full amount of pressure. Keep under pressure for about 30 to 60 seconds or more depending on quantity of material.

Pressing naked bud often requires cleaning the rosin, which means repressing and filtering after collection. To refilter rosin, chill it until the stability allows you to place it inside a bag — no more than 7 or 10 grams at a time. Repress the rosin at 200˚F degrees and ease into the pressure slowly. Note: this can be a slippery sticky mess.

PARCHMENT PAPER OR PTFE SHEETING

No matter what approach to rosin tech you choose, parchment paper IS absolutely essential. That's parchment paper — NOT WAX PAPER. Make sure the paper you choose doesn't have any coating. It is available in cooking supply sections of most supermarkets. One strong low-cost option many rosin extractors use is Costco brand.

PTFE "paper" (a nonstick plastic sheeting made from polytetrafluoroethylene) is increasingly used in the packaging of concentrates as an alternative to parchment paper, and in some instances it can be used as an alternative for pressing rosin as well, but only when lower pressure is being used. PTFE is OK to use for pressing hash rosin, but not to press flower, which requires higher pressure, because the sheeting stretches, making collection difficult.

MACHINE PRESSING FLOWER

Pressing buds yields between 10 and 35 percent — roughly corresponding to the cannabinoid content of the starting material. If a strain tests around 25%, expect a yield of about 25% of the material's weight in rosin under optimal conditions. An ounce of buds yields about a quarter ounce of rosin.

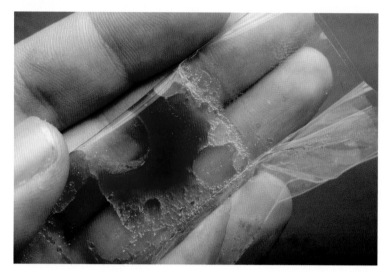

BHOgart Terp Proof PTFE paper is non-reactive. Unlike silicon-coated parchment paper, it will not disintegrate into botanical oils, damaging your extract.

Before pressing, make sure the moisture level in your material is just right: too low and your yield and quality will suffer, too high and your rosin will be difficult to collect or will smell and taste like chlorophyll and may even turn green.

Most rosin extractors heat the material 150° to 250°F range. This varies based on the material's moisture content, which also affects yield. Always check yields and rosin quality at different temperatures to determine the best setting for a particular batch. Once you have a batch dialed in, you'll be able to use the setting, or combination of settings. One significant temperature, 220°F, is the decarboxylation point of THC.

Start at the "ceiling" (250°F and work your way down in 5 or 10-degree increments, taking note of your quality and yield at each step. It's best to start at 250°F to determine the maximum yield for that strain. Most likely, the quality and color of the rosin will be compromised by that high a temperature. There's lots of variation between strains and presses when it comes to yields and temperatures, which is what makes this "dialing in" process so crucial to ensuring quality end product and sustainable yields.

Lowering temperature usually results in higher quality, but this is not always the result. However, lower temperatures will reduce yield, sometimes drastically. It depends on both the quality and the "personality" of the starting material. Always start high and work your way down, doing about 3 to 4 test presses to dial in the strain.

Make sure to be consistent with the amount being pressed. Spread the bud so it forms an even layer. For example, if pressing 7 grams, use 3.5 big buds and 3.5 smaller buds. Remove all stems from flowers. This will result in tastier rosin. Conversely, buds with stems or seeds creates a less satisfying extract..

Once stems are removed and flower is weighed to the desired amount, using a bag opening tool to keep your bag open, place two small buds in first and make sure that they're packed into the corners tightly. This prevents loss of oil to the corners. Once they're packed, fill the bag with the remaining material evenly with no voids and an even thickness of between one quarter inch and a half-inch, leaving a one-inch flap for a fold. There will be two additional corners after the fold; fill these voids to ensure even flow and prevent loss.

Always cut and fold parchment paper prior to filling; ripping parchment in the middle of a job is messy, awkward, and inefficient. Place the parchment paper evenly into the press. Make sure to center and place the packed rosin bag between the layers of parchment paper. Press the material about halfway to allow the heat to transfer through it. Wait five to 15 seconds, depending on the amount being pressed. This process is referred to as "preheating" as it allows the trichomes time to become viscous.

Once the trichomes have melted, apply full pressure. You should start to see oil flowing from the platens. Depending on how fast the extraction is happening and amount being pressed, keep pressure on the material for 35 to 90 seconds. The reason for the time variation is that flow rates vary by variety and freshness. Slow-flow flowers require pressure and heat for a longer period. Fresh flowers with fast-flowing oil should be pulled off the heat quicker.

A good way to judge how long to keep the bud under pressure is to watch the color of the oil and the degree to which it's flowing. Once the flow starts to darken and slow down, it's time to pull. You can also press without the use of a bag, using a pre-press or just pressing buds as is. A press allows you to press more material in a smaller surface area, creating more pressure to larger amounts of material.

Left: Lifting paper set up in the press.
Right: Filled rosin filter bag placed in a press. Photos: Sasquash

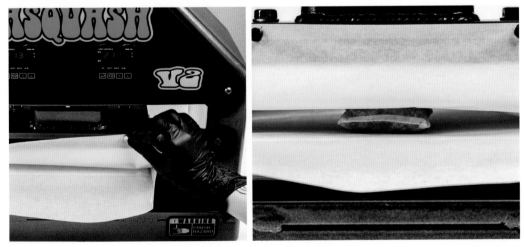

MACHINE PRESSING HASH AND KIEF

Top-shelf rosin that rivals the flavor, potency, and aesthetics of BHO often starts as high-grade bubble hash. Five-star hash can already be pressed into a dabbable consistency using only light manual pressure, but the application of rosin tech has pronounced effects on the clarity and color. As with flower, start with well-cured starting material with no moisture or mold.

Use temperatures from 150°F to 210°F, as with flower, start at the "ceiling" and work your way down in 5 or 10-degree increments, taking note of your quality and yield at each step. Test the material at different temperatures and find a happy medium between quality and yield. The lower the yield, the more refined the product.

This process is a bit trickier than pressing buds, but it will ultimately produce the most valuable product. The higher the oil content of the starting material, the quicker and higher the yield will be. But if you use hash or sift that's green with plant material, you need to treat it the same as bud. Some sift and hash gets overwashed or tumbled, which means that it might require top-temp (250°F) pressing.

Pack the bags no thicker than a quarter inch when pressing hash or buds. Make sure to pack them evenly. Don't overpack them. If the material is packed too densely, it will expand and can tear the bag. This results in a sticky mess of fabric and half-melted hash and a tedious clean-up.

You should also pre-press the hash inside the bag to prevent expansion and bag blowout.

Once the bag is packed evenly and the parchment is ready, center the hash on the press within the parchment paper, allow the platens to meet the material and wait about 25 to 45 seconds, allowing the trichomes to melt and become viscous. Remember to always ease into the pressure with about an 8th of an inch movement at a time, waiting in between movements for about 5 to 10 seconds.

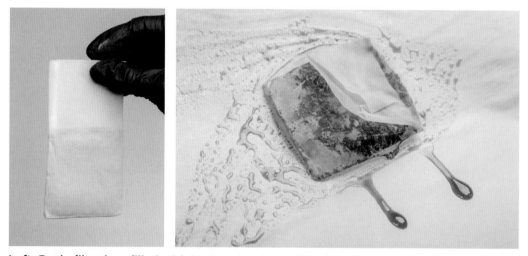

Left: Rosin filter bag filled with hash, ready to fold the top over and press.
Right: Pressed hash with rosin around it. Photos: Sasquash

Oil should start to ooze out the sides immediately. Once platens meet and oil stops flowing, apply a bit more pressure to the remaining plant material to filter any remaining rosin out of the plant material — you don't need to apply any more than 5000 psi when finishing a hash press.

A hash press could take up to five minutes to complete, depending on the temperature and melt factor of the starting material. Expect yields to come between 40 to 70 percent, and upward of 90 percent or more if using five-star, full-melt, fresh-frozen hash. If hash or sift is green and full of plant material, expect the yields to come in closer to flower —10 to 35 percent.

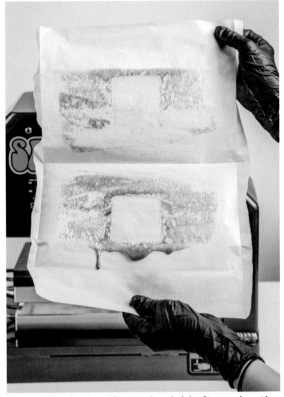

Displaying the rosin yield after using the Sasquash press. Photo: Fred Morledge

REPRESSING FOR SOLVENTLESS THCa

After collecting rosin, you can re-press it to filter the THCa. It's an easy 2- to 3-step process using low temperature and 35 micron filters. First, fill 35 micron bags evenly with rosin. Set your temperature to 150°F. Much like re-pressing rosin for naked-press cleaning, ease into your pressure slowly with 8th inch movements at a time. A high-terpene, dark oil will flow out of the bag. A white powdery substance remains in the bag. It is mostly THCa. You'll return between 25 to 50 percent THCa, depending on potency and grade of starting product.

After collecting the THCa in the bags, pack the THCa evenly into another 35 micron bag and wrap with an additional 35 micron bag. Press this material at 170 degrees, same as before, ease into pressure, and this time there won't be a flow. The additional bag was added to soak up any remaining residuals that may have been left in the THCa. The THCa is white powder and a little difficult to handle. It can be pressed again at 230 degrees to make it more stable and glassy. Place all THCa powder in another 35 micron bag and re-press at 230 degrees, always slow and with ease. The last step will ooze and should yield close to a 100 percent return.

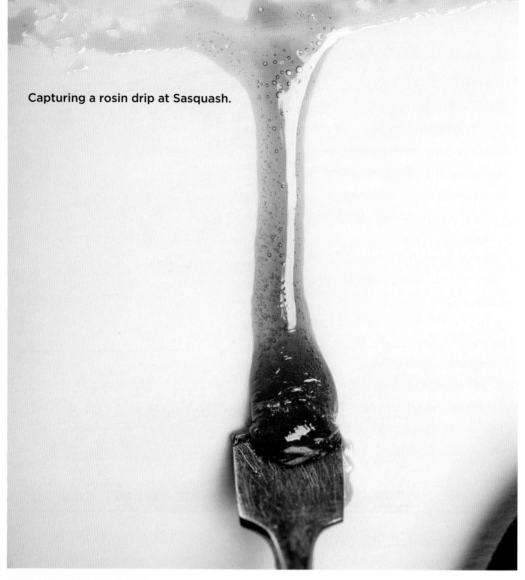

Capturing a rosin drip at Sasquash.

COLLECTING ROSIN

Gathering up rosin after pressing is often more challenging than the press itself. Depending on the starting material, moisture, temperature, and timing, a wide range of consistencies can result. It can be a stable, easy-to-gather material or a sticky sap. Hash rosin will be more stable (less sticky and gooey) than flower rosin, which is often difficult to gather.

No matter what consistency you're working with, it's probably best to work in as cold a room as possible, ideally with cold work surfaces, to increase or maintain the rosin's stability while you collect and package it. Make sure you wear gloves to prevent contamination of your rosin with skin oils and to avoid getting rosin stuck to your hands. After pressing out the rosin, leave all the papers in the refrigerator for about five minutes to cool everything down and stabilize the oil. Cold plates or cold blocks can be used to help with collection — an aluminum plate left in the refrigerator is an ideal cold surface.

Avoid scraping parchment paper, as this could result in paper particles being scraped into the final product.

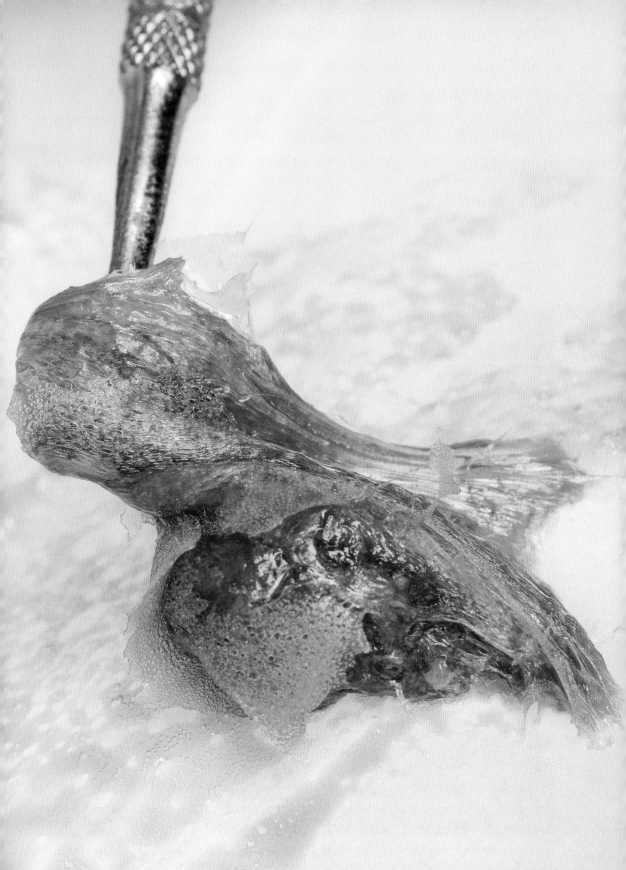

Collecting rosin after pressing at Sasquash. Photos: Fred Morledge

CURING AND STORAGE

After collecting the rosin in a ball, there are different ways to cure it. Forming a large ball is a good way to protect most of it from oxidization and to prevent the evaporation of terps.

Always store rosin in sealed containers in the refrigerator. The refrigerator will preserve terpenes and prevent oxidization. If you don't plan to weigh it out, leave in a large ball inside a sealed container.

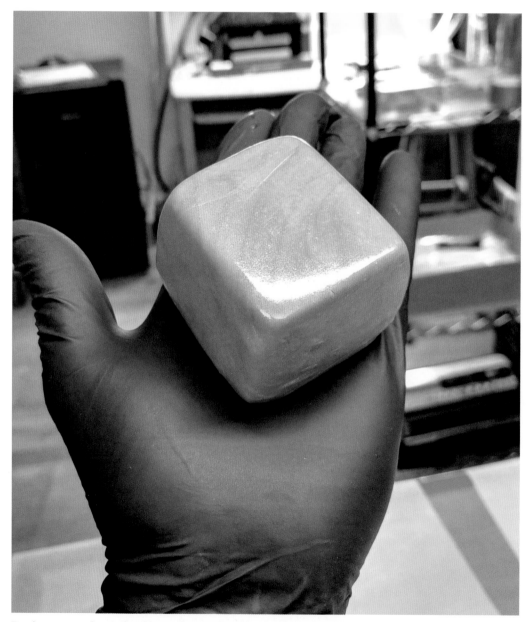

Rosin square from the HoneyButter Rosin company in Mendocino is made from select organic genetics and made with moderate temperatures for shorter duration pressing.

Most rosin will show its consistency instantly. Depending on temperature, the rosin will either stabilize, budder up, or turn to crumble. If you notice the rosin is becoming budder directly out of the press, it's a good sign that the entire batch is going to turn to crumble. If it's not buddering up in the press, there's about a 50 percent chance of it staying shatter.

Most rosin can be converted into crumble by using the "taffy pull" method.

THE TAFFY PULL METHOD

Taffy pulling is exactly what it sounds like. Just as taffy is pulled to change the consistency of the candy, pulling and twisting the rosin transforms the consistency from a liquid state to a dry consistency.

Taffy pulling could take upward to four or five sessions of pulling. Once rosin becomes more of a peanut butter consistency, you know it's ready to package. Work in a cold room, weigh out half-gram chunks, and roll them into balls. Then, with no heat, smash the balls between parchment paper to desired thickness and allow the rosin to dry before putting it in a sealed container.

Before putting in the effort to alter the appearance of the rosin, make sure there's a demand for the consistency being pursued. Taffy-pulled rosin is more desirable to some dabbers, but others like the shatter consistency.

Taffy from the Honeybutter Rosin company starts by procuring the highest quality starting material as possible.

SHO Products

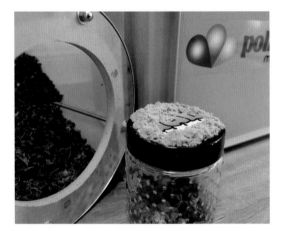

In the early days of Silicon Valley, groundbreaking products were often born in 2-car garages, where budding entrepreneurs employed geeky wisdom, elbow grease and spare computer parts to ply their trade. This same DIY ethic is an integral part of the cannabis community, where new technology is starting to radically transform the way people manufacture and consume a plant that's been around for thousands of years.

In early 2015, the founders of SHO Products learned about a new solventless extraction method called "Rosin Tech", which involves applying heat and pressure to cannabis. This technique allows producers to extract cannabinoids and terpene rich oils from the cannabis plant without the use of harmful and sometimes toxic solvents. At the time, most people were using and breaking hair straighteners, and it was clear there was need for equipment designed specifically for making rosin.

In typical start up fashion, SHO Products took its idea from concept to market. Working out of garage, we developed and released Rosin Tech Products, the first full line of rosin presses to hit the market. Filling a void in the marketplace, the business grew rapidly. Shortly thereafter, SHO Products acquired a 15 year old brand and line of dry sift tumblers known as Pollen Masters.

In 2016, SHO Products acquired a provisional patent for a new rosin manufacturing process using two heated rollers instead of two heated plates. Dubbed the Rosin Roller, this technology is being further developed to increase production times while limiting the amount of time the oil is under heat and pressure.

With a continually expanding product line, SHO Products has become a leading distributor of ancillary products in the industry. Whether you're a large producer looking for commercial grade rosin presses, dry sift tumblers, bubble washing machines and freeze dryers, or a consumer who needs an electric nail for an enhanced dabbing experience, SHO Products has you covered.

SHO Products continues to educate consumers about the benefits of solventless extraction.

We host the Solventless Experience (check www.solventlessexperience.com for our next event) at Cannabis Cups all around the world, allowing consumers to make their own hash oil and learn about the medical benefits of the cannabis plant. The company has won top honors more than 15 times and now has 300+ domestic and international retail stores.

In addition to our industry leading solventless extraction equipment, we have launched the world's first dab shop for the concentrate connoisseur. After years of seshing with dabbers around the world, comparing experiences with various concentrate tools and accessories, we launched DabNation.com.

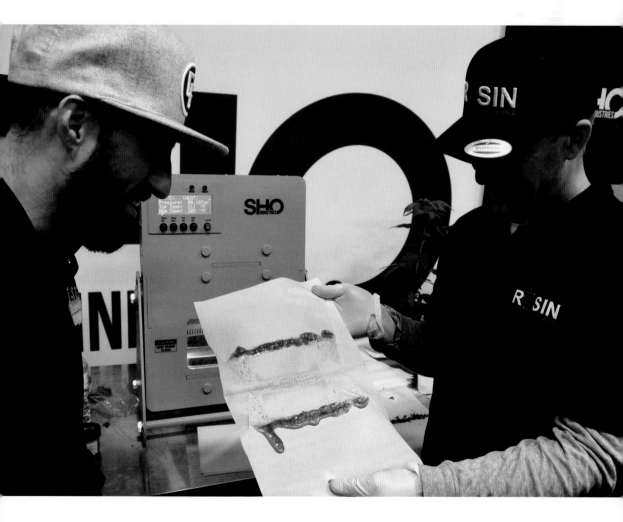

Gourmet award-winning Lucky Lemon Cookie by Derby Bakery contains white chocolate chips and tastes sweet and zesty. To keep the cannabis flavor to a minimum it is infused with THC oil from organic cannabis.

CHAPTER 9

Edibles

Eat Me, Drink Me — This Chapter Makes You Higher

In her best-selling cookbook published in 1954, Alice B. Toklas revealed a recipe for "Hash Fudge," which is similar to the Moroccan enhanced edible "Mahjoun." This may have been the first published recipe for a cannabis edible. After that, edibles grew steadily in popularity. Now their popularity is growing logarithmically, and they are especially appealing to the new wave of people coming to cannabis for both medicinal and adult use.

At first the common carrier was a fudge brownie. But the recipes list soon expanded. Now there are so many food infusions available to consumers, purchasing from a dispensary can sometimes feel like selecting from a buffet line: sweet, crunchy, savory, medicinal.

GLOBAL EDIBLES

Eating cannabis is a practice embraced by so many societies and cultures across the globe that it's probably easier to just single out regions that don't have some historical tradition of cannabis medicine — Antarctica springs to mind. Cannabis tinctures and salves were once mainstays of holistic healing across the globe, before the advent of state and national prohibition in the early 20th century, following the global cannabis prohibition created by the United Nations' Single Convention on Narcotic Drugs in 1961.

To find one of the earliest recorded uses of cannabis edibles as medicine, we have to reach back over 4,000 years to the birth of Traditional Chinese Medicine. According to ancient historical records, around 2700 BC, Emperor Shen Nung of the Xia Dynasty — one of China's three "Celestial Emperors — composed "The Herbal," a foundational text of Chinese medicine still used with modifications by contemporary TCM practitioners. For this contribution, Shen Nung is often referred to as the "Father of Chinese Medicine."

India has a global reputation for its charas, but its cultural connection to cannabis is also deeply rooted in bhang, a sweet, milk-based beverage used in traditional Ayurvedic medicine and one of the earliest cannabis edibles. Before the adoption of American taboos around its use, bhang consumption was much more common, and the drink is still a central feature of the Holi festival and other Hindu religious observances. The drink — a mixture of pulverized cannabis flower, clarified butter or ghee, milk and Indian spices — is particularly prized for its appetite-stimulating and sleep-inspiring effects.

BHANG LASSI

Bhang Lassi is the traditional Indian beverage for Holi, the Hindu celebration of spring, but it's imbibed all year round. A curd-based drink flavored with sugar and spices, it can also be made with yogurt and milk. You can make a Bhang Lassi at home with canna milk or some hash or kief.

In India, Bhang Lassi is prepared by mixing a bhang ball (typically a blend of oily hash and finely ground dried bud) with hot milk that has usually been infused with almond paste, a bit of coconut milk or butter, and some ginger, saffron, or other spices. Vendors, like chefs, have their own recipes using different combinations of spices. This is my recipe. Experiment based on your own taste.

- 1½ cups yogurt/curd, chilled
- ½ cup canna milk
- 4–8 teaspoons sugar to taste
- ½ tsp cardamom powder (optional)
- 1 pinch saffron (optional)
- 1 pinch garam masala (optional)
- 1 tsp rose water (optional)
- 1 tsp of almond paste, chopped almonds or pistachios

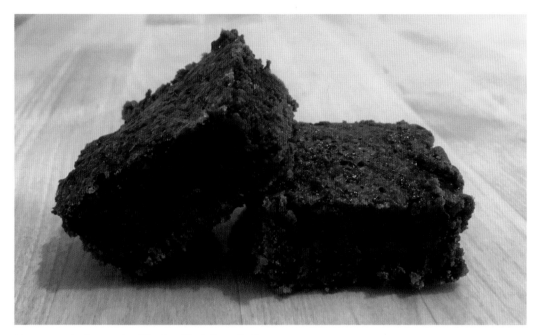

Homemade brownie. Photo: Christian Petke

BROWNIES

Ingesting cannabis was once the primary mode of consumption in the United States. In the 19th and early 20th centuries, people relied on over-the-counter "tonics" that were often cocktails of folk medicines and powerful narcotics, derogatively described as "snake oils." Cannabis confections such as "Hasheesh Candy" were openly advertised in magazines like *Vanity Fair*, and sold in the Sears & Roebuck catalog as a remedy for "anxiousness" and other ailments. At the same time, pharmaceutical companies were manufacturing cannabis tinctures. The crackdown on "snake oil" treatments and the federal prohibition laws enacted in 1937 put a temporary end to edibles in America. In the face of prohibition, Americans adopted the Mexican practice of smoking raw cannabis flowers because the cigarettes were easy to prepare, took little equipment, and were easy to hide. We've been doing it ever since.

Brownies are the perennial favorite and remain the stereotype for all edibles; but why the brownie? The short answer is Alice B. Toklas and her cookbook. Brion Gyson, a Beat poet, contributed his recipe for "Haschich Fudge" to *The Alice B. Toklas Cook Book*. However, this ancestor of the modern magic brownie didn't actually contain any chocolate; it was made from spices, nuts, fruits, and cannabis.

It wasn't until the 1968 release of the film *I Love You, Alice B. Toklas,* starring Peter Sellers, that pot brownies as we now know them first exploded into the mainstream consciousness. The movie piqued the interest of the general public, reduced the stigma of eating cannabis, and framed it as an opportunity for an adventure.

After the movie, brownies took hold as the preferred method for eating cannabis. One reason might be that the rich chocolate flavor masked the less tasty plant flavors. Practically every person who's eaten cannabis at some point in their life has tasted a pot brownie.

"Magic brownies" were still largely perceived as a novelty item in the United States, generally reserved for festivals, parties, and other occasions for celebration. There was no "dosing" in those days; you just ate some, waited, ate some more, and sometimes ended up taking a longer, stranger trip than anticipated.

Brownies also played a central role in San Francisco's medical cannabis revolution, which planted the seeds for Proposition 215 and the dawn of a golden age for medicinal cannabis. Mary Jane Rathbun earned a hallowed space in cannabis activism history (and the moniker "Brownie Mary") for her groundbreaking activism, which began when she started providing cannabis-infused brownies to AIDS patients at San Francisco's General Hospital at the peak of the AIDS crisis. From then on, cannabis edibles became a cornerstone of California medical cannabis, providing potency and discrete consumption for those who can't or simply don't smoke buds.

BEYOND BROWNIES

Brownies were just the beginning. Any food item you can think of is likely to exist in a cannabis-infused form, from potato chips to chicken wings. In this new age of cannabis acceptance, edibles are no longer just something college kids furtively scarf while standing in line for festival tickets; they're also part of an expanding salon culture focused on the intersection of gourmet cuisine and ingested cannabis.

As the world of cannabis edibles grows larger in both scope and focus, the demand for specialty products that cater to specific dietary needs and culinary trends is creating a new discussion around the marriage of food and cannabis. Breaking bread has always been a foundational element of any culture, and cannabis culture is no exception.

The American cannabis culture of the late 20th century viewed edibles as a ticket to adventure and excitement, but with a new set of laws, the early 21st century has seen the rise of a more holistic, health-minded perspective regarding the use of edibles. Instead of eating a 100 mg cookie and zoning out for hours, people are increasingly drinking 5–15 mg of cannabinoids in their cup of tea with breakfast and perhaps chewing a 10 mg stick of gum on the subway on the way to work. New cannabis users are looking to enhance their daily life with cannabis.

New regulations regarding potency limits on edibles, including potency caps on edible portions, such as the 10 mg dose cap imposed by California's regulatory framework, are changing the way people ingest cannabis. New regulations on manufacturing facilities ensure quality, consistency, and purity. Because of this, a professional edibles culture has emerged, which has drawn capital into various sectors of the edibles market. Just a few decades ago the notion of a commercial cannabis product was considered absurd; there was no real demand for such a

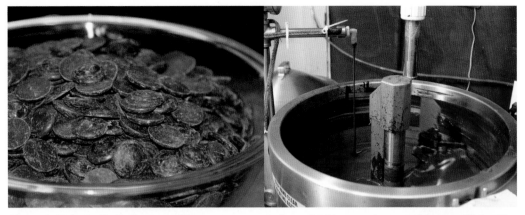

Chocolate in bulk, before melting.

Automated tempering machine heating, stir-ring, and circulating the melted chocolate.

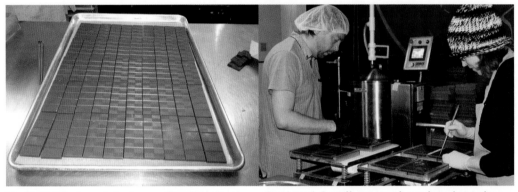

Medicated chocolate bars after being re-moved from the refrigerator and molds.

Paul and Candi move chocolate into the corners of the chocolate bar mold while it's on a shaker, assuring consistent dosing and even chocolate throughout the bar.

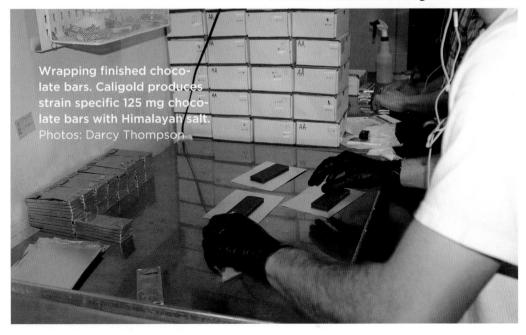

Wrapping finished choco-late bars. Caligold produces strain specific 125 mg choco-late bars with Himalayan salt.
Photos: Darcy Thompson

Heavenly Sweet makes a wide range of baked and non-baked edibles including their Cookies & Cream Treat and their Rainbow Treat, both 100mg.

thing and nobody was making it. Now, cannabis product marketing is beginning to mirror wine and fashion industry trends. In this new market, companies are required to put more effort into branding, packaging, and placement.

THE SCIENCE BEHIND WHY THAT BROWNIE RUINED YOUR NIGHT

There is a vast and expanding body of research that supports the broad physiological benefits of responsible cannabis consumption and confirms the numerous effective applications of cannabis medicine. And while clinical research is absolutely crucial to further standardize and understand the mechanisms at play, the fundamental efficacy of medical cannabis is a matter of scientific fact.

Humanity's trust in cannabis medicine stretches across millennia: Hundreds of thousands of generations of human beings agree — cannabis medicine works. And though there are undoubtedly distinct medical benefits and applications for inhaled cannabis, particularly concentrates, much of the human history of cannabis medicine has been characterized by people ingesting it. Why? Because of cannabis metabolites.

Most cannabis users, even those with elevated tolerances, report that eating cannabis edibles provides a more intense, longer high than smoking or dabbing. The reason for this is simple: Eating cannabis edibles actually does provide a more intense, longer high than smoking or dabbing.

One of the main benefits of edibles over smoking (apart from the obvious health benefits of not setting plant matter on fire and pulling the smoke into your lungs) is that ingested cannabis is metabolized by your liver before entering the bloodstream, which transforms its chemical makeup, producing THC metabolites, namely 11-OH-THC. This metabolite is more potent than regular THC (Delta-9THC), and while it's created in the body when cannabis is inhaled, the levels of 11-OH-THC can be over 10 times higher when it's ingested.

THC'S JOURNEY — FROM ACID TO METABOLITE

Many people still use THC as a catch all when discussing the potency of buds, as in "this strain generally tests around 23 percent THC." But from a technical standpoint, the cannabis plant doesn't actually produce THC, not the delta-9 THC people are thinking of when they say THC. It actually produces THCa, the precursor acid to delta-9; the process of decarboxylation converts the acid to the "active" delta-9 form, which is itself converted to the THC metabolite 11-hydroxy-THC, which metabolizes into the brain more quickly than delta-9. The final stage of THC's journey is the conversion of 11-hydroxy-THC to 11-Nor-9-carboxy THC, an essentially inert secondary metabolite that possesses an exceptionally long half-life, which is why it's the primary target of most blood- or urine-based cannabis drug tests.

The effects of an edible on the human body are different for each individual. It depends on several factors including weight, experience, hydration, recent food intake, and overall liver condition.

Processing cannabis isn't especially taxing on the liver, so consuming edibles while taking pharmaceuticals isn't necessarily a no-no — it will depend on the individual's tolerance as well as the particular medication. Depending on one's digestive system, it can take up to 90 minutes for edibles to take effect, so always wait a while before consuming more. Use moderation, especially when taking pharmaceutical drugs that cause drowsiness.

CBD edibles can provide many benefits without the intoxicating effects of THC. There are also some people who claim benefits from juicing and consuming raw cannabis, which provides THCa and other raw cannabinoids that won't cause intoxication. Many incorporate raw cannabis and hemp plant into their diet specifically for this reason — to be able to reap the positive effects and advantages of cannabis without experiencing the high.

DOSAGE GUIDELINES

From *Marijuana Herbal Cookbook,* by Tom Flowers

For a person weighing 150 pounds who has some experience using marijuana, a single edible dose is in the following range:

Marijuana leaf: 1/2 to 2 grams **Sinsemilla:** 1/8 to 1/2 gram

Average bud: 1/4 to 1 gram **Kief** and **hashish:** 1/8 to 2 grams Using these guidelines, 1/4 ounce makes the following number of servings:

Marijuana leaf: 4–15 servings **Sinsemilla:** 8–34 servings **Average bud:** 8–25 servings **Kief** and **hashish:** 4–34 servings

You can see that these are rough guidelines. The reason is that the potency of bud, kief, and hash varies so much. Smoking the material before cooking with it helps gauge its strength. People's tolerance levels also vary.

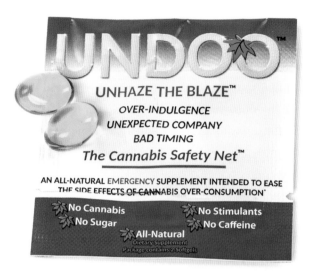

UNDOO™ softgels are the only patented Cannadote, formulated to ease the discomfort of too much THC. UNDOO™ softgels are also effective for a tolerance re-set.
Photo: Fred Morlege

RESPONSIBLE CONSUMPTION

Most people find that eating 5 to 20 mg of decarboxylated cannabis provides the desired effects, so the average edible "dose" should probably fall somewhere in that range when producing for the public. If you're making a tray of brownies at home however, dose it to your personal preferences.

As adult-use legalization rolls out in several states, one main concern brought up by both proponents and opponents of cannabis is accidental ingestion by children. Although the actual danger presented to a child by cannabis has been radically overstated (often to the point of sensationalism), there is a broad desire to keep cannabis out of childrens' hands, and much of the regulation aimed at edibles is motivated by that desire. As the general public continues to gradually embrace medical and recreational cannabis, it falls to the industry and community to support proper education to the new users.

Here's a list of basic rules to follow for getting the most enjoyment (and the least trouble) from your edible experience.

ED'S TEN EDIBLE RECOMMENDATIONS

1. **Pace Yourself**

   The key to a good edibles experience is the same as the key to good barbeque — "low and slow." Start with a low dose of 5 to 10 mg of THC and wait at least an hour (the effects can take anywhere from 30 minutes to two hours to kick in, depending on the person) before consuming any more cannabis. Your digestive system processes cannabis slowly, and if you've eaten prior to having an edible it can take up to 2 hours to feel the effects. After that time has passed, if you still don't feel the desired effects, then feel free to eat a little more of your edible.

2. **Label Your Edibles**

    If you make your own edibles (or if a friend shares anything with you), always label and store all infused products properly. Labeling is especially crucial for avoiding accidental ingestion: Cannabis can't harm you, but accidentally eating a hash-infused granola bar before that big job interview may not work out in your favor. It's easy to forget what is and isn't medicated without labels, and if you don't know the precise potency, you can at least write "mild" or "strong" on the label — anything that increases your ability to make an informed dosing decision at a later date.

3. **When Mixing Bud and Booze, Know Your Limits**

    When you ingest an edible it goes through your digestive system, is broken down, and then heads to your liver, where THC metabolites are formed. Alcohol is also processed through your liver, and the additional effort of processing both substances at the same time can be too intense for some people. Always practice moderation when you drink, but when you combine alcohol with edibles, make sure you practice even more.

4. **Beware of Edibles on an Empty Stomach**

    Edibles are much more intense when consumed on an empty stomach. That's not necessarily bad, but you need to make sure your actual nutritional needs are met before piling on cannabinoids. Be sure to eat a solid, nutritious meal before taking your infused edible.

5. **Do Not Operate Heavy Machinery (or Any Machinery)**

    Obviously this means your car, but please consider not operating any machinery at all whatsoever. A bicycle doesn't qualify as "heavy," but if you try to ride one in traffic, in the grips of a high-dose edible, your chances of survival are greatly reduced. Just take it easy. Stay in a safe place where you will feel in control at all times. Do not drive, and make your surroundings calm, relaxed, and enjoyable.

6. **Do Not Allow Pets or Minors to Access Edibles** (If you are a minor, please wait a few years before consuming edibles.)

    As noted previously, there are worse things in your home that your pets and kids can get into. The chocolate in an infused brownie is more harmful to your dog than the cannabis, and no child, regardless of age or weight, is going to die from eating cannabis. That said, letting kids and pets eat your edibles is socially irresponsible and, let's be honest, a total waste of good edibles. If you have young children in the household, lock your cannabis products out of reach from little hands or paws.

7. **Keep Other Weed-Free Food Handy**

    Make sure you have something to eat at all times, particularly when you've eaten an edible. Hunger can strike suddenly, and it's best to have a snack and not need one than need a snack and not have one.

8. **Try to Stay Hydrated**

    "Cotton mouth" is a plague no person should have to experience, and like most things in life, the key is prevention. If you stay hydrated from the start, you'll never experience the shrieking panic and agony of being too parched to speak and too high to get something to drink.

9. **Do Not Give People Edibles Without Their Permission**

    Here's a golden rule you can apply to your entire life: Don't do/give things to people without their informed consent — period. Apply this to edibles and you're good. That means never deceive somebody by giving them infused food without their knowledge or giving them a higher dose than they think they're getting. It can be psychologically distressing to experience acute intoxication when you didn't plan for it or aren't used to it. Don't be "that guy;" let people make their own decisions about what they want to put in their body.

10. **Don't Panic**

    Always keep that timeless bit of all-weather advice from *The Hitchhiker's Guide to the Galaxy* in mind; Don't Panic. If you feel that you've overindulged with your edible ingestion, then you're already ahead of the game; you've recognized the problem. Remain calm, drink water, and try to relax — reminding yourself that you'll be fine and that this state is temporary usually helps. Find a quiet place where you can lie down, listen to soothing music, or just sleep it off. Some people claim a dab of CBD shatter or certain vitamin formulations can "undo" an intense high, but the only 100% effective method is time.

MAKING YOUR OWN EDIBLES

From Ancient China and India, the history of humanity's love affair with eating cannabis reaches back millennia. Hundreds of generations of human beings agree: Ingested cannabis has major health benefits. So when you cook up a batch of something with a little something extra from the garden, you're linking into a chain that stretches across an ocean of human history. What follows is a selection of basic recipes and processes that will have you cooking up your stash in no time. Keep in mind, these recipes represent the basics—juices, oils, butters, and honey can all be used to infuse other dishes. There is now a wealth of high-quality cannabis cookbooks on the market for those who want to take their culinary efforts to the next level. See the selected reading section in appendix for a list of cannabis cookbooks we recommend.

COOKING WITH FIRE: PREPARING CANNABIS TO INFUSE EDIBLES

Without heating it up or decarboxylating it, "raw" cannabis is full of nonpsychoactive THCa — it's actually considered a "superfood," leading some people to eat or juice and drink it raw to access the over 400 distinct chemical compounds inside the plant, including vitamins, essential oils, and nutritional acids. "Fresh green juice" may not be instantly appealing to every taste, but it's a quick, efficient way to get the nutritional and anti-inflammatory benefits of fresh vegetables and raw cannabis.

DECARBOXYLATION

1. Preheat an oven to 140˚F (60˚C). If you have an oven thermometer to gauge your oven's true temperature, that's even better.

2. Break the leaf or bud down into more manageable pieces, and place on a cookie sheet as if toasting spices. Do not overload the cannabis so that the pieces are on top of one another.

3. Place in the oven and monitor for 30–40 minutes (depending on oven strength and strain of weed). You're looking for a golden-brown color as opposed to the more vibrant green of the untoasted leaf.

4. Take out of the oven, allowing the toasted cannabis to cool. Then place it in a food processor and pulse it for a second so that it becomes coarsely ground.

5. Prepared this way, the cannabis may be used for cooking in various recipes.

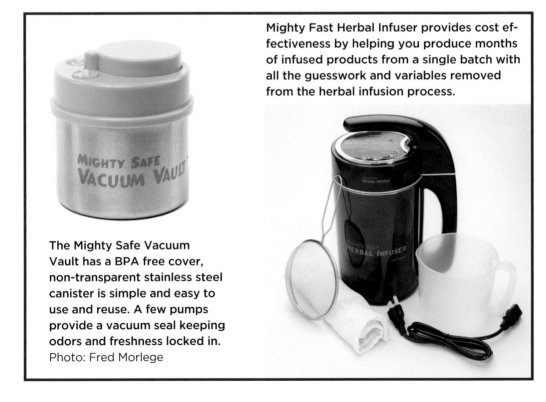

Mighty Fast Herbal Infuser provides cost effectiveness by helping you produce months of infused products from a single batch with all the guesswork and variables removed from the herbal infusion process.

The Mighty Safe Vacuum Vault has a BPA free cover, non-transparent stainless steel canister is simple and easy to use and reuse. A few pumps provide a vacuum seal keeping odors and freshness locked in.
Photo: Fred Morlege

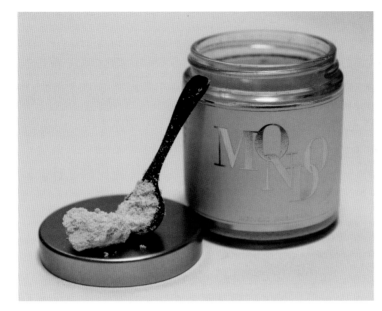

Mondo Powder was developed as a low calorie, all natural, THC powder that dissolves instantly and can be precisely measured.
Photo: Darcy Thompson

USING HASH, KIEF, OR TINCTURES IN FOOD

While this chapter focuses on using leaf and trim material to make ingredients, hash, kief, and hash oil are easy-to-use, excellent ingredients for cooking. They concentrate the cannabinoid dose without the vegetation, resulting in a cleaner, less "green" taste.

Not much concentrate is needed for each portion, making it even more important that these ingredients are mixed thoroughly to keep portions uniform. Alcohol and butane solvents remaining from processing hash oil evaporate quickly when exposed to cooking heat.

Hash, kief, and hash oil need some preparation before they're used in cooking. Grind, shave, or chop the hash to a fine consistency using a coffee grinder or blender. Then add cooking oil or alcohol and blend into a mush or slush using a blender or by placing everything in a jar with a tight cover and shaking it.

Tinctures are ready to consume so they can be dropped (added to food using a dropper) on baked goods, salad dressings, beverages, or other foods shortly before serving. Make sure to measure dosage because it's easy to overdo the drops, and they're more potent than cannabinated alcohol, butter, milk, or oil.

USING EXTRACTS IN RECIPES

Clear distillate and other active cannabis extracts can also be used in place of butter. One benefit is that the infusion can be done after the food is prepared, allowing individuals to decide their own dosage. This is especially beneficial when attempting to infuse entrées and other dishes being shared by several people. Because using active oils is as simple as squeezing some onto your plate, we haven't dedicated much space here to recipes using them. However, clear distillate can certainly be used to infuse beverages and other items outlined below.

JUICING

Many people juice raw marijuana for its health benefits. Juicing fresh buds and leaves lets you ingest large amounts of THC in its nonpsychoactive acid form, THCa, and CBDa, the acid form of CBD, which has anti-inflammatory, anti-oxidant, and cancer-fighting properties, as well as stimulating effects on the immune system. The juice also contains terpenes, which have mood-altering and therapeutic qualities. It doesn't produce the high of decarboxylated bud, but the terpenes produce noticeable effects.

The therapeutic potential of raw cannabis has not been studied in clinical trials, but reports of individuals achieving good results, such as Dr. William Courtney's wife, Kristen, who, suffering from Lupus, improved dramatically after treatment with the raw juice. Dr. Courtney recommends using it in large quantities, as much as 100 times greater than you would smoke. Many other people also report medical improvement for a variety of chronic physical ailments. Effects may be immediate or take weeks of treatment. Drinking large quantities of marijuana juice as a dietary supplement may be rough on the kidneys and gallbladder, so it's not recommend for people with conditions affecting those organs.

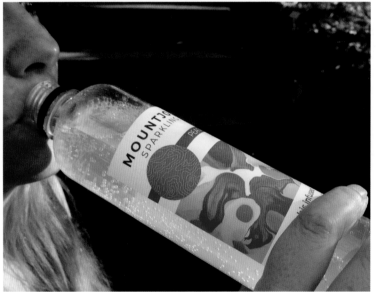

Mountjoy Sparkling Cannabis-Infused Sparkling water is fast acting, convient, zero calories and made with organic cannabis. 10 mg THC in every 16 oz bottle. Photo: Darcy Thompson

Commercial juicing devices such as wheat grass juicers are the most efficient. Juice is made by dropping fresh-from-the-plant bud, trim, and leaf in the blender, then straining it using a sieve or squeezing it through cheesecloth to eliminate the drained vegetative material. If you are not averse to alcohol, soak the solids in grain alcohol or high-proof vodka, then squeeze it out to remove the remaining cannabinoids. The juice tastes bitter, so most users mix it into other drinks.

Soaking leaf or bud in water removes dirt or other environmental elements from the plant surfaces. Check the material for mold and mildew. Without the heat of cooking or combustion to inactivate them, these unwanted materials flow with the juice.

You can preserve the juice by freezing it. Fill ice cube trays with your fresh juice, freeze it, then use as desired.

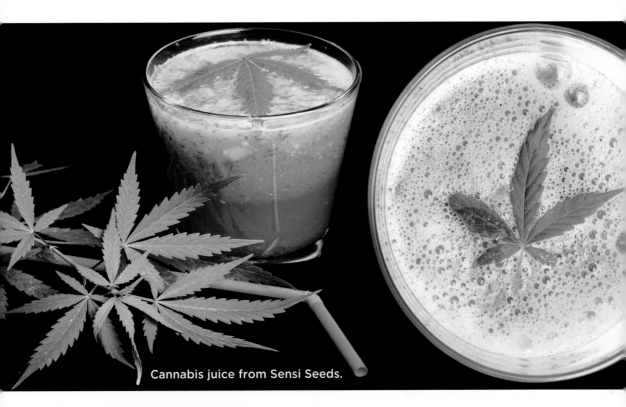

Cannabis juice from Sensi Seeds.

FRESH GREEN JUICE RECIPE

While we might be imbibing special brownies for their "special" qualities, when it comes down to it, we're still eating a brownie. If that habit starts adding up and you're looking for a healthier alternative, you can try this simple green juice recipe. As with any fresh, home-squeezed juice, you can add or remove ingredients based on your personal preferences.

Ingredients:

- 5 cups of spinach or some other mild, leafy green
- Two cups of kale or rocket greens
- 7–10 large cannabis fan leaves
- 1 large apple
- 1/2 a cucumber
- 1/2 a lemon

Preparation is as simple as putting everything in a blender and pressing a button.

Juicing is great for the full-spectrum benefits of raw cannabis, but if you're looking for the benefits of active cannabinoids, you'll need to either use a cooking method that is hot enough to decarboxylate your cannabis ingredients or pre-decarb your material to convert the cannabinoid acids into active cannabinoids. Some concentrates are already active, but if you choose to work with flower, trim, or leaf, you'll definitely need to decarboxylate the cannabis first.

CANNABIS TEA

Marijuana teas are common folk medicines used for upset stomachs of children and adults in Jamaica. Cannabinoids are weakly soluble in hot water, so making a tea by boiling buds, leaf, or trim in water will not extract much of them. The heat and agitation of boiling knocks some of the cannabinoids from the leaves. They float loose in the water. Many of the pigments and terpenes that give marijuana its color and flavor are water soluble, so the tea takes on a pleasing color and aroma and has a mild psychoactive effect. Adding dry lecithin granules, which are emulsifiers, helps the cannabinoids mix into the tea.

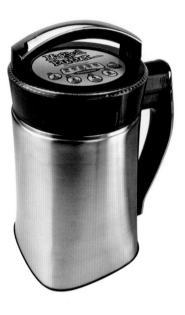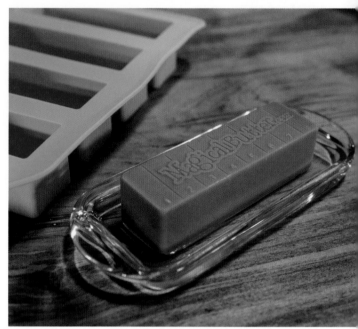

Left: The MagicalButter® machine is the world's first countertop Botanical Extractor™ and was designed for infusing herbs into butter, oil, grain alcohol, and lotions.
Right: A stick of MagicalButter® just out of a mold.

BUTTER ME UP

Butter and oil are perfect for cannabis baking, sautéing, and infusing because cannabinoids are oil soluble. There are many ways to make cannabutter and infused oil, as well as relatively inexpensive machines that make it easy for anyone to make cannabis-infused butter, oil and even milk in one container, in one step. But if you don't have these implements to assist your infused cooking, here's a simple recipe to make infused butter, olive oil, and coconut oil.

Butter is a popular choice, but olive and vegetable oil are versatile and generally considered more nutritious. Coconut oil is particularly beneficial as it metabolizes quickly. This not only means quicker onset of effects, but also faster evacuation from the body, which some users feel prevents or reduces the severity of cannabis "hangovers." Cocounut oil also has a milder taste, which makes it more versatile than other fatty cannabinoid mediums.

Over-the-Stove Method: Infusing Butter, Vegetable Oil, Olive Oil, and Coconut Oil

Ingredients:

    1 cup of ground cannabis flower (or less for milder potency)

    1 cup of oil or butter of your choice

You'll need:

    Strainer or cheesecloth

    Grinder works best or an appliance like a food processor, blender, or coffee grinder to pulverize the cannabis. Once again, not too small of a grind, as it can result in too much plant matter in the oil.

    Double-boiler, slow cooker, or saucepan

Directions:

1. Grind the cannabis with a food processor or blender, but not too small, as anything too small will go through the strainer. You may include the entire flower, leaf, and trim, depending on your preference.

2. Combine oil and cannabis in your double-boiler or slow cooker, and heat the two together on low or warm for at least 4 to 6 hours. This allows for the cannabis to be decarboxylated and activate the THC in the cannabis. Low and slow will add to the potency of the infused oil, but if you heat too high, it will destroy the THC content. Stir occasionally throughout the process. If on the stove top, a small amount of water can be added to the mixture to help avoid burning.

3. Once the infusion is completed, let it cool down and then strain in a strainer or cheesecloth. Do not squeeze the cheesecloth; this will simply add more plant matter to your oil. All remaining plant material can be discarded or used in other dishes. The oil's shelf life is at least eight weeks and should be refrigerated.

NOTE: Be cautious when using the oil to prepare dishes that require heating. Do not microwave and choose low heat whenever possible. Whatever method you choose, temperature of the oil should not exceed 245°F.

    Start out low and slow; five to ten milligrams of THC in one dose of an edible is a safe starting point.

Medicated olive oil by Pot D'huille contains a ratio of one mg THC per 1 ml olive oil. It can easily replace butter in any cooking medium or be drizzled on to pizza, pasta, soups and more.

Pot d'Huile

CANNABIS FLOUR

Ground marijuana can be substituted for a portion of the flour in a recipe. Bread made with whole wheat and hempseed flour with finely ground marijuana has a pleasant, savory taste. When used as a replacement for flour, dried marijuana should only be used in a ratio of 1 part ground leaf material to 2 parts regular flour to maintain a good texture and taste.

To turn leaf or bud into flour, simply grind it thoroughly in a clean coffee grinder. If the plant material is in pieces too big for a grinder, run it through a food processor or flour mill first. After grinding, use a flour sifter to ensure that your marijuana flour has a consistency much like wheat flour.

Preparing marijuana flour with butter, margarine, or oil makes it even more effective and can be used to replace the flour and part of the oil or butter in a recipe. This method converts the THC acid to THC, dissolves cannabinoids into the butter, and eases digestion.

SWEETS: SIMPLE SYRUP, HONEY AND CANDY

CANNABIS SIMPLE SYRUP

With edibles many of us are seeking ways to add an infusion into our diets that's easy and simple. A "Cannabis Simple Syrup" could be just the thing to add to almost any drink or edible. Simple syrup is a breeze to pour into ice tea, hot tea, coffee, water, lemonade, a smoothie, a cocktail, or even over ice cream or yogurt. The best aspect of this is that simple syrup is so easy to make. If you can make a can of soup, you can make simple syrup.

Ingredients:
 3 cups of filtered water
 3 cups of fine granulated sugar
 2 tablespoons of vegetable glycerin (you can find this at your local health food store)
 2 grams of finely chopped cannabis leaves (not too fine or straining will be challenging)
 A jar, bottle, or some other container with a lid on it
 Strainer and/or cheesecloth

1. Place the water and sugar into a pot and bring to a boil and stir until the sugar is fully dissolved.
2. Once the sugar has dissolved and the mixture is boiling, add the cannabis. Cover the pot and let it low boil gently for 20 minutes. During this time is when the decarboxylation will occur. This step will assist in releasing the THC in the flower into the liquid. But make sure that you don't allow it to get too hot or boil over.
3. After it boils for 20 minutes, reduce the heat. Add the vegetable glycerin and let the entire liquid simmer for 5 to 6 minutes.

4. Take off the heat and allow to cool down and strain the cannabis leaves from the liquid.

5. Now pour the strained clear liquid into a clean container.

This simple syrup is fully activated and ready to infuse any beverage with sweetness and a cannabinoid kick. If you're feeling a bit adventurous, it also serves nicely in cocktails that call for simple syrup or sugar, but make sure you use either cannabis with a mild flavor or something that will accentuate your beverage.

SWEET HONEY RELIEF

Bees are the only insects that are able to manufacture a food that may be eaten by humans. This incredible product, honey, is the only food source that contains all of the vital enzymes, vitamins, minerals, and water that is able sustain life. Honey has been respected for its medicinal values for thousands of years. It is well known to have properties that can assist in wound care; and it is anti-bacterial, has anti-inflammatory properties, and even heightens memory sustainability. It's no wonder that we would want to incorporate the two sources together and make a perfect combination of medicinal and fortifying blends to build a healthy immune system with cannabis and honey.

Adding cannabis to honey creates a powerful and healthy natural remedy, since both are known to have healing antibacterial and anti-inflammatory properties. Cannabis-infused honey can be used topically or ingested — depending on the desired effects. Infusing honey has been practiced for over 3,000 years and is an extremely versatile material with a large number of healing properties. When you add various herbs, you're creating a powerful combination that can prevent and fight illness and diseases in the body.

CBD may be effective at elevating support to one's immune system and suppressing influenza viruses. So who wouldn't want to sit back with a cup of tea infused with honey that would not only relax you but also strengthen your immune system with the properties of cannabis. Any cold or flu season would be improved with cannabis honey integrated in afternoon teatime.

Making infused honey is very simple, and once it's done, you may freeze or refrigerate it and store for months. Honey requires a fat to bind to. We recommend adding a bit of coconut oil to assist in binding the cannabis and honey in a cohesive sweet nectar. Or if you have a cannabis tincture, it is even simpler to add to honey; no heat or straining you just add the drops to the honey, mix well, and your cannabis honey is ready to enjoy.

For the culinary aficionados, here is your place to be creative with additions to your honey. Let your palate guide your way with blends of herbs, spices and flowers to make flavorful infused honey. You'll be amazed by how much a sweet herb–flavored honey can boost a special sauce or dish. You can add dried lavender, chamomile, sage, rosemary, thyme, vanilla, or cinnamon to your satchel of decarboxylated cannabis. Or you can make a big batch of cannabis

honey tincture and then make a bunch of different flavors by infusing them all separately. Also, you can add the infused honey to body topicals such as scrubs, lip balms, body butters, lotions, salves, face masks, soaps; the list is endless.

This honey and cannabis tincture is effective because the cannabis has already been decarboxylated, which requires an extra step before infusing your honey. If you want a less psychoactive tincture, you can skip the decarboxylation process and go straight to the slow cooker step. Follow the instructions in the recipe on decarboxylating in the edibles chapter.

You'll need:

Cheesecloth or strainer

Crock pot or slow cooker

Spatula

Jar to hold 16 oz with lid (mason jar is perfect)

Ingredients:

12 oz honey

1/8 gram of cannabis

1/4 cup coconut oil

Directions:

1. Add warm water to a crock pot and set on low. Place jar with honey and cannabis in jar. Have enough water to immerse jar up to where the honey is on level at.
2. Set the slow cooker to low. Honey may simmer a bit, but should never come to a boil. Check your mixture periodically and switch the slow cooker to warm or off if it gets too hot.
3. Keep the heat on for 6–8 hours. Turn off the crockpot and let the mixture sit until cool or overnight.
4. Pour the honey through cheesecloth or strainer, squeeze the cloth to get every last bit of liquid out, combine coconut oil and honey till well blended.
5. Pour honey into sterilized mason jars. Refrigerate or freeze for longer shelf life.

Keep a bit of honey at room temperature for adding to teas, coffee, and smoothies, but you can kee a container in the refrigerator where honey can be stored indefinitely. Add a little sweetness to your life that adds to your health!

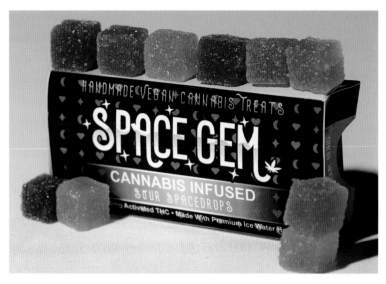

SpaceDrops are handcrafted vegan gummies made with organic ingredients, including premium ice water hash from Talking Trees Farm. Produced in Humboldt County, each drop is 10 mg THC and come 10 to a box.

CANNABIS HARD CANDIES

The infused hard candy has been an intro for many into the world of edibles. The ease of a sucker or small hard candy with a bright fruit flavor has been the beginning of a love affair for candies that have a satisfying and long effect. For most people, hard candies take longer to consume and so the psychoactive effectiveness is prolonged. The variety of flavors offers more opportunities to experiment; just be aware of the dosing. Here's a simple recipe on infused hard candy.

You'll need:

Saucepans, one medium and one large

Scissors

Candy thermometer

Candy molds for a Jolly Rancher size or something similar. If you don't have this, you can just pour into a canna buttered sheet pan. But that makes dosing difficult to judge. If you have a sucker mold and sucker sticks, that works better.

Ingredients:

1/4 cup Infused tincture

2 cups granulated sugar

2/3 cup light corn syrup

3/4 cup water

1/2 teaspoon lemon emulsion

1 teaspoon superstrength fruit flavor of your choice

5 to 10 drops of food coloring depending on the flavor to match the color. (Red for cherry etc.)

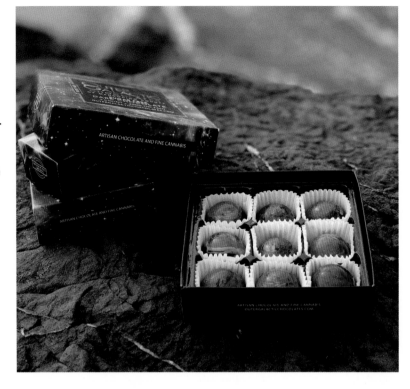

Crafted in Mendocino County, Outer Galactic Chocolates are made with chocolate sourced from small sustainable farmers and are hand painted. Dark, milk or dark sugar free, they contain THC distillate for quality and consistency.
Photo: Lizzy Fritz

Directions:

1. Put your tincture in a smaller nonstick saucepan and heat on low. Cook until almost all of the alcohol has evaporated (about five minutes). It should look like molasses.

2. Add emulsion and flavoring extract to complement the flavor of candies you want to make. Then stir.

3. Remove from heat and let cool for five minutes.

4. Mix sugar, corn syrup, and water together in a large saucepan and stir on medium heat until sugar dissolves.

5. Insert candy thermometer, making certain the thermometer doesn't touch the bottom of the pan. Bring mixture to boil without stirring.

6. Continue to cook the mixture without stirring until the temperature reaches 260°F. Add food coloring and do not stir. Continue to cook until thermometer hits 300°F.

7. Remove from heat precisely at 300°F. Add flavoring and tincture reduction and stir quickly.

8. Quickly pour into prepared molds and let sit at room temperature for 5 minutes.

9. Wrap or store in containers. If your tincture was a certain amount of milligrams, divide it by how many Jolly Ranchers you made, and that will be the THC milligram count in each piece of candy. Remember go low and slow until you know your personal dose!

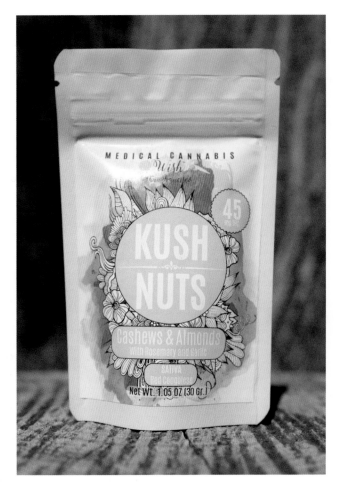

Kush Nuts is a savory edible free of added sugars and artificial ingredients. Kush Nuts are a blend of cashews and almonds infused with premium quality cannabis.

FOOD ADVENTURES

As you explore the world of cannabinated food, here's a list of suggestions:

- Light foods and snacks are the best match when looking for recipes to cannabinate.

- Flavor extracts, particularly orange extract, seem to neutralize cannabis odors. Just add a teaspoon to any cookie or cake recipe. Orange extract imparts a nice fruity flavor to baked goods and is good with chocolate. Orange extract can also be used when making marijuana butter or oil.

- Strong spices such as ginger, cinnamon, cloves, or nutmeg mask the smell of marijuana when making baked goods. A teaspoon of any of these spices added to cookie recipes blends well with the taste of marijuana leaf. Chocolate also helps neutralize the smell of marijuana and disguises any green coloration.

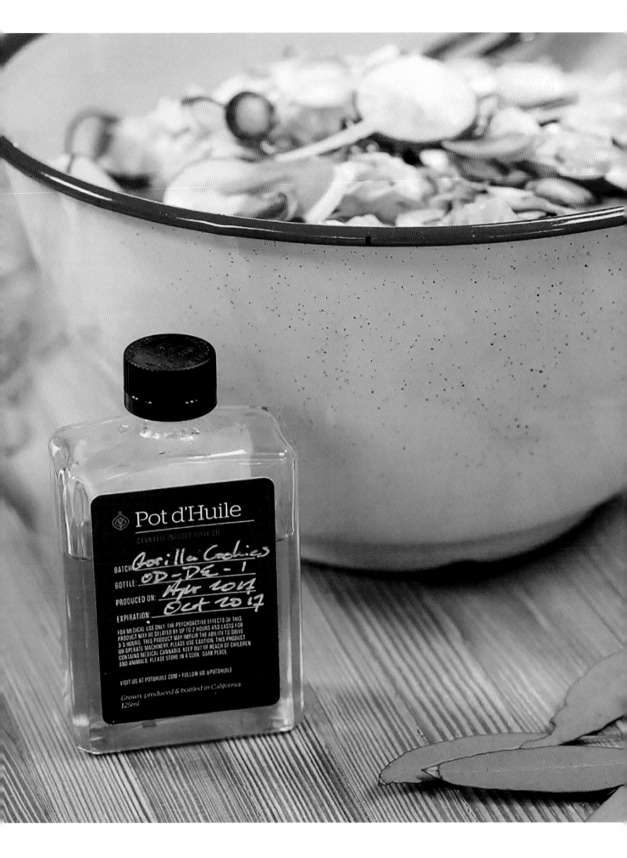

Soothing cream by Mermaid Wizdom absorbs quickly replenishing and protecting skin. It contains 200 ml of CBD in a two oz container.

CHAPTER 10

External Cannabis Medicine:
Topicals and Transdermals

M ost cannabis consumption methods involve getting cannabinoids inside your body, usually via the respiratory or gastrointestinal organs. But cannabis medicine can also be applied directly to your largest organ — the epidermis; the top layer of skin that stretches over the outside of your body. Cannabis infused topicals were once a mostly homemade phenomenon, but they have become a distinct pillar of the growing cannabis marketplace, with companies offering infused lotions, balms, oils, transdermal patches and various other products that can be absorbed into (or through) the skin for relief of pain, soreness, and inflammation.

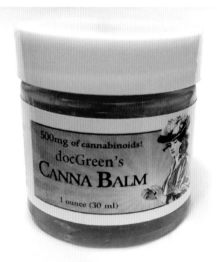

Canna Balm from Doc Green's is their strongest most potent topical with over 500mg of active cannabinoids per jar. Made with pure, raw, solventless CO2 concentrate, bee propolis and pollen, as well as essential oils for increased healing.

Skin is the human body's first line of defense against the elements and potentially harmful microbial contaminants, but this huge organ (roughly 20 square feet all told) is also involved in several crucial physiological processes like detecting and regulating body temperature and circulation, sensing pain and other vital stimuli, and retaining or expelling moisture. The epidermis consists of four to five layers of tissue that encompass various glands, ducts and membranes, all of which have distinct physical processes that allow them to function properly. Like the rest of your body, the efficiency of these processes can be directly improved by activating the homeostasis regulating mechanisms of the Endocannabinoid System (ECS). In addition to CB1 and CB2 receptors, skin cells contain enzymes responsible for endocannbinoid metabolism. So the skin essentially contains its own version of the ECS, and that system plays a very important role in skin physiology.

TOPICAL OR TRANSDERMAL?

Because many of the ECS receptor sites are located in the epidermis, cannabis infused "topical" products are applied directly to the organ being targeted; the skin. But skin is semi-permeable, which means cannabinoids can also be absorbed into your system through your skin — this is called "transdermal" application, which is often achieved by using a transdermal patch. Because topical applications of cannabis, like balms or liniments, absorb into the epidermis and don't breach the blood-brain barrier, they have no psychoactive effect. In contrast, transdermal products use the skin as a conduit to the bloodstream and depending on the dosage and formulation may make you feel "high."

TRANSDERMAL APPLICATION

With transdermal application we're seeking to impact systems beyond the epidermis. Transdermal therapies are able to pass through the skin and target muscles deep below the surface, decreasing inflammation and thereby pain.

No matter what the end result is, the goals of transdermal treatments are to get the active ingredients into the body while bypassing the first pass metabolism of ingestion and provide prolonged, steady dosing unavailable from inhaled therapies. Transdermal administration provides a direct route to the bloodstream, supplying the whole body with active cannabinoids, and offers continual release of the drug over time so dosing can be less frequent than other routes of administration. Transdermal patches contain large amounts of cannabinoids mixed with solvents that increase the permeability of the outer layer of skin. They are also discreet, allowing patients more control over their preferred dose. The biggest disadvantage of transdermal cannabinoid delivery is the same as for any transdermal drug; the difficulty of designing formulations to get the drug through the skin. Certain compounds such as alcohol, amines and terpenes interact with the lipid matrix of the skin to alter its structure and allow for increased drug penetration. Use of low currents, ultrasound and microdermabrasion are also effective transdermal methods, though much less frequently employed.

Transdermal patches like those designed by Cannabis Science and Mary's Medicinals are available in many states where medical and/or recreational cannabis is legal.

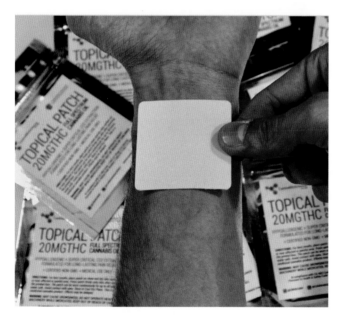

Cannabis Science transdermal patches deliver a specific dose of medication through the skin and into the bloodstream promoting healing with a controlled release of medication.

TOPICAL APPLICATION

With topical applications we're seeking a localized effect, meaning we're trying to cause a physical reaction in the immediate area of skin being treated by reducing inflammation and pain sensation. Additionally, topicals have been shown to be effective in treating a multitude of skin conditions such as melanoma, dermatitis, skin tumors, acne, psoriasis and itchiness from bug bites or rashes. But because the skin has direct physical and neurological connections to every other organ in the body, topicals provide unique benefits when used as the application point for cannabis to treat issues that aren't just skin-deep.

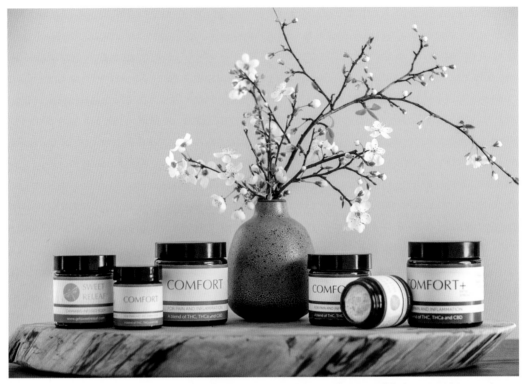

Sweet Releaf's body butter is infused with pure trichomes from multiple cannabis strains, cold harvested to preserve full potency.

For example, somebody suffering from a strained muscle in their back doesn't have a "skin condition," but that doesn't mean an application of pain-relieving ointment to the area of skin covering and surrounding the injured muscles won't provide relief, particularly when taken in conjunction with an orally ingested and/or inhaled cannabis remedy. In fact, this is one of the most efficient and effective general strategies for using cannabis medicine, particularly for pain; pinpoint the source of the pain, use topicals and inhaled cannabis for immediate impact and edibles or tinctures to secure lasting relief.

A WORD ON THE WORD "NONPSYCHOACTIVE"

Generally speaking, external applications of cannabis aren't psychoactive. Topical applications stay within the epidermis and never cross the blood-brain barrier, but transdermal applications do reach the bloodstream, meaning those with high enough doses of active cannabinoids could potentially induce mild euphoric impacts.

For most people, external applications of cannabis won't provide the euphoric effects of inhaling or ingesting cannabis. That said, many people do experience a mild "high" when using external applications, even those that don't penetrate the bloodstream, which is likely an endorphin response to the physical relief of reduced or alleviated pain.

HOW CANNABIS INFUSED TOPICALS WORK

As covered in a previous chapter, humans are biologically primed to reap the benefits of phy-tocannabinoids, which supplement our own naturally produced endocannabinoids. When we consume cannabis, a network of receptors crackles with activity, kick starting biochemical reactions that can alter everything from blood pressure and pain response to appetite and skin barrier function.

Cannabis-infused lotions, salves, oils and sprays work by binding to the CB2 receptors of the ECS that are located near the skin. The absorption rate for cannabinoids is quite low, particularly for THC, while CBD and CBN are absorbed at a higher rate.

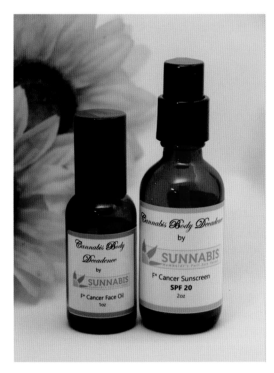

F* Cancer Sunscreen and F* Cancer Face Oil by Sunnabis are infused organic, Humboldt sun-grown cannabis with vitamin C and essential oils.

For targeted healing, there is a range of topical products to consider. For example THC and CBD have been shown to reduce inflammation in cases of psoriasis, eczema, and allergic dermatitis. They can help regulate sebum production and moisture retention within skin, and clinical trials have shown positive effects of topicals on acne and seborrheic dermatitis. Hemp oil (containing high-levels of CBD), cannabis-derived CBD and THCa-based products, are gaining popularity as skin remedies. Hemp oil is a common ingredient in many anti-aging cosmetic products created to protect and also heal damaged skin.

We find that at least a small amount of THC will "activate" the CBD, making it more effective, so to get the full effect you might consider a product with both THC and CBD.

Different topicals have different benefits to offer depending on the way they are processed and the ingredients that are used, so experiment with various topical and transdermal products to see what works for you. Some carrier agents are more effective than others at penetrating the epidermis. Other additives such as calendula and comfrey offer increased healing properties by further lowering inflammation and increasing analgesic effects.

THE BENEFITS OF EXTERNAL CANNABIS MEDICINE

The commercial and cultural explosion around external applications of cannabis is an example of how new modes of consumption are revolutionizing perceptions of cannabis as improved accessibility, safety and efficacy move cannabis medicine further into the cultural mainstream. Groups such as athletes and seniors who have traditionally been adverse to cannabis consumption are increasingly benefitting from non-psychoactive topicals. Your grandparents will want to join the green wave when they see how topicals provide relief without altering their sensory perceptions.

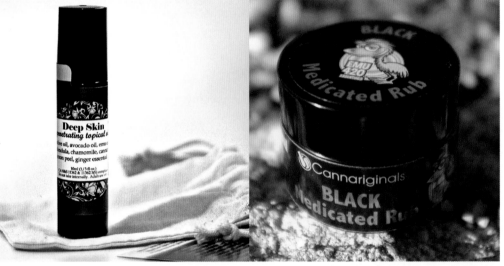

Newell's Botanicals Deep Skin Topical Oil absorbs quickly and completely delivering cannabinoids to affected tissues and was formulated to be effective on skin damaged by the sun and arthritis.

Cannariginals EMU 420 Black Medicated Rub will help you relax. Its high cannabinoid content makes it perfect for pain-relief and the pure emu oil carrier delivers transdermal effects. Cannariginals also produces a mentholated product which provides a cooling effect.

Arthritic pain caused by inflammation can be effectively treated with products that have THCa and CBDa, both of which are anti-inflammatory. Active THC is not as effective for treating inflammation, but is thought to be more effective on pain not associated with inflammation.

Cannabis topicals are made with material extracted from the plant in a variety of ways using solvents like CO_2 or Ethanol to produce oils, cooking down the buds and leaves, or cold harvesting the trichomes (crystals) without processing them.

MAKING YOUR OWN TOPICALS

These topicals recipes are made with an infused coconut oil, which there is a recipe for in the edibles chapter. But you would be fine to use olive infused oil as well.

Capsule and roll-on production at Kind Medicine. Photos by Darcy Thompson and Arya Campbell

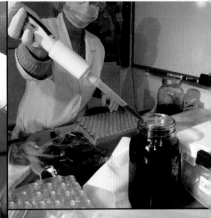

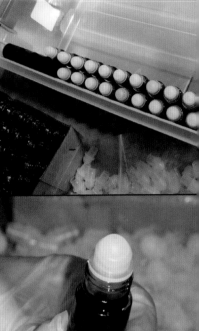

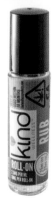

Kind Medicine Roll On's are a CBD 1:1 ratio and are great for healing, calming and moisturizing the skin, as well as helping with nerve pain.

Cannabis Balm Recipe

First of all, clean and disinfect your area of topical preparation. Your space should be uncluttered and wiped down with a disinfectant with all your tools, containers and utensils set out. You will need a double boiler, measuring cup, measuring spoons, whisk, mixing bowl, spatula, mixing spoon, paper towels for cleaning up spills.

In a double boiler heat the water to a slow boil. Add in:

1 Cup infused coconut or olive oil

¼ Cup Olive Oil (Organic is best)

1/3 Cup Beeswax

Whisk intermittently until beeswax is melted. Once melted you may add in essential oil for scent such as peppermint, lavender or tea tree oil. Pour mixture into a bowl and let cool. During this time you may whip it to have a smoother consistency. While still slightly warm you may transfer into containers to finish cooling, then cover and store in a cool place. Make sure your containers are clean and sterilized as well.

Cannabis Lotion Recipe

This is the same as making a balm, but when the everything is melted and taken off the heat from the double boiler add in:

1 Cup aloe vera gel

1 teaspoon vitamin E oil

2 tablespoons shea butter or cocoa butter

If you would like an enjoyable scent to your lotion, this is the time to add in a essential oil of your choice.

If you like a more fluid lotion you may add in more E oil or olive oil.

Arthritis Balm or Lotion — If you suffer from arthritis or muscle, tendon pain you may add 1 teaspoon of cayenne powder to your batch of balm or lotion. Mix well and make sure that when applying you keep away from eyes, mouth and noses. Wash hands immediately after applying.

Headache Balm — If you find that you have a headache or sadly suffer from migraines, you'll find that a topical may assist in releasing the painful issues. Add in essential oils of eucalyptus, peppermint, lavender, tea tree oil to your coconut and beeswax mixture once you've taken it off the heat. Depending on how strong you would like the balm 12 to 18 drops. Balance the scents so they blend together well. Once completed you may apply lightly to your temple and at the back of your neck for the best results. Also, it's nice to take a warm towel and infuse with your balm and place on your forehead or back of the neck.

Relaxing Sleep Balm — After taking off the heat you may add dried lavender flowers or dried rose petals or both and these should be a fine chop on the flower blend no more than 1/8 of a cup. You may add in 5 drops of chamomile oil as all of this ad to relax the mind and body for a better relaxing restful sleep. Rub a small amount under your nose, temples, hands and feet. Then laydown, relax and have sweet dreams.

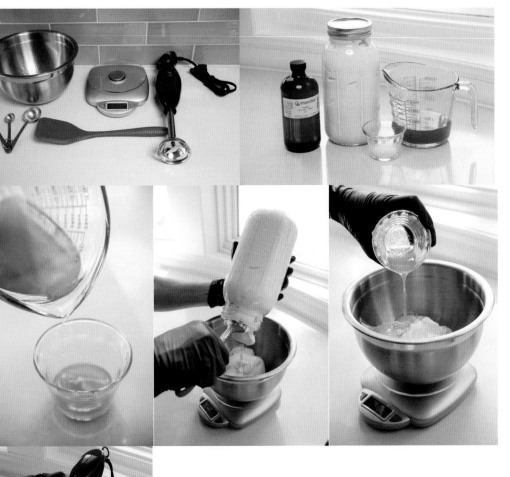

Top: Basic supplies needed to make infused cannabis lotion including coconut oil, lotion, and tools to mix and measure.

Middle – Measuring infused cannabis coconut oil, base lotion, and combining them.

Bottom – Thoroughly mix the lotion and infused oils. Mermaid Wizdom.
Photos: Fred Morlege

SPA PRODUCTS AND BEYOND

THE CANNABIS SPA EXPERIENCE

Beauty and spa products infused with cannabis oils are a wonderful way to address health concerns while pampering yourself. Top manufactures of beauty and wellness brands are just beginning to understand the promise cannabis-derived ingredients hold for anti-aging products. As this end of the cannabis market continues to evolve, here are a few elements of the cannabis spa experience to look for in your community.

Ganja Yoga: Most major cities where cannabis is legal (either medical or adult use) offer ganja yoga classes—sometimes called 420 yoga or elevated yoga. Many people find integrating cannabis into their yoga practice encourages a quieting of the mind and an increased ability to focus on their practice. Many dispensaries and cannabis collectives host classes focusing on meditation, yoga, acupuncture, acupressure, Pilates, massages and holistic counseling, reiki, qi gong, tai chi, and more.

Cannabis Spas: In addition to the ubiquity of yoga, cannabis spas are also popping up across the country, catering to a clientele interested in beauty and wellness. Dispensaries have long capitalized on the link between cannabis and health, naming their companies with spa-like names. Today, in most major cities, you can find massage therapists who offer CBD and THC infused oil massages. LoDo Massage Studio in Denver, for example, offers a "Mile High Massage," infused with THC, CBD, arnica, juniper and peppermint oils.

Cannabis Tourism: Bud and Breakfasts and cannabis spas are a fairly new phenomenon in the United States; thankfully, foreign countries offer spa opportunities as well. In Jamaica, Coral Cove Cannabis offers weddings and honeymoons with spa treatments on site. The Rastafarian Church provides gift baskets to guests upon arrival.

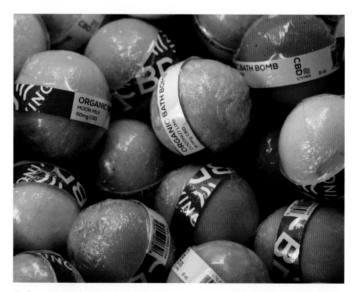

Take your bath to the next level: Fill up the tub, drop in CBD Living's Bath Bomb and lay back and enjoy the lovely color and fragrance. Each bomb weighs 8 ounces and contains 60 mg of CBD. Fragrances include Coconut Lime, Eucalyptus, Lavender and Amber Bergamot.

Whether or not a cannabis spa experience is within reach, wellness enthusiasts can always incorporate infused therapeutic products into their in-home beauty routines. Get ready to breathe deeply and relax as you find your green spa experience.

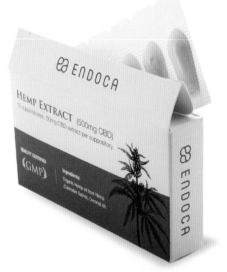

Endoca receives regular feedback from our clients and found that many people who have difficulties swallowing, find their suppositories an effective way to bypass oral consumption and still feel the benefits of CBD. Each suppository contains 50 mg of CBD and is made using organic raw CBD extract (containing both CBD and CBDA) and coconut oil.

VAGINAL CANNABIS

Vaginal and rectal cannabis products are a new area of interest for cannabis researchers. A range of cannabis lubricants and suppositories hit the market around 2014 and were marketed primarily as a sexual stimulant. Today, many women swear to the effectiveness of these products in treating everything from menstrual pain endometriosis, migraines, fibromyalgia, hemorrhoids, back-pain, and sleeplessness. There are many advantages to internal administration of cannabis. The bioavailability of THC and CBD through vaginal or rectal absorption is over twice that of absorption through the gastrointestinal tract. Internal membranes are highly absorbent and effective in transporting and distributing cannabis around the body; whereas when we take cannabis products sublingually, a portion of the medication is lost as it passes through the body.

Empower® 4PLAY is a light, fresh, pH balanced cannabis-infused sensual oil, designed to enhance arousal and intensify pleasurable sensations during sex. Women also use 4PLAY when they experience menstrual cramps.

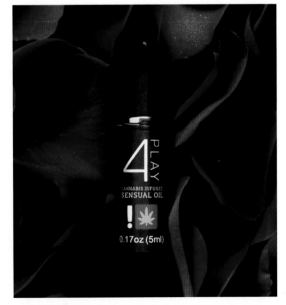

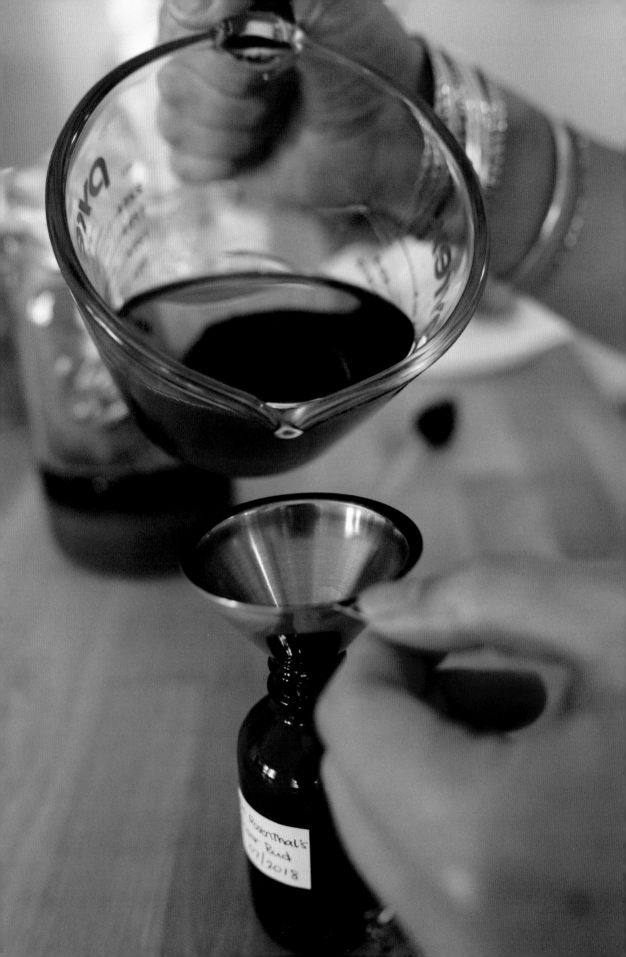

CHAPTER 11

Tinctures, Capsules and Beyond

TINCTURES

Before cannabis prohibition, tinctures were the most common way of buying and consuming marijuana in America. Recently, they've been making a comeback. Commercially prepared tinctures are now available in dispensaries in many states. Tinctures are discreet to use and are quite easy to make at home.

A tincture is a concentrated extract of any herb in liquid—usually alcohol, oils like medium-chain triglyceride (MCT) oil, or sometimes glycerin—that is taken by mouth as a drop on or under the tongue. Alcohol is used to separate the cannabinoids, terpenes, and other essential oils from the marijuana plant material and acts as a preservative. In herbal medicine, tinctures are commonly 25% alcohol, which is achieved by diluting the mixture with water. People who do not want to consume alcohol may opt for glycerin or oil-based tinctures.

Methods of making alcohol tinctures vary from extremely simple and low tech to complex distillation apparatuses that produce highly purified cannabis oil. The easiest way to make tinctures is an alcohol soak. All that's required is a bottle of 100 proof or higher drinking alcohol and cannabis leaf, trim, bud, or kief. Add the cannabis to the liquor, let it soak for at least a week, then strain (or not) and enjoy.

CHOOSING THE ALCOHOL

No matter what type of marijuana is going into the tincture, starting with a quality solvent is important. The purest grade alcohol is USP medical-grade, 190 or 200 proof neutral grain spirits. It is available from laboratory supply companies.

More commonly available is 190 proof Everclear brand alcohol, which can often be found at liquor stores. Note that Everclear is marketed in two strengths: 150 proof (75% alcohol) and 190 proof (95% alcohol). Get the 190 proof. Sale of Everclear 190 proof is currently banned in California, Florida, Hawaii, Iowa, Maine, Minnesota, New York, Nevada, Ohio, and Washington.

An alternative high-proof option that is available in some of those states and online is an extremely pure form of Polish vodka called Spirytus that comes in at 192 proof, or a percent purer than Everclear. Polmos Spirytus, Spirytus Rektyfikowany, and Baks Spirytus are some of the brands that can be found in the United States.

If these purified options are unavailable or you are interested in a little flavor (not for smoking/vaporizing), other high-proof liquors can be used.

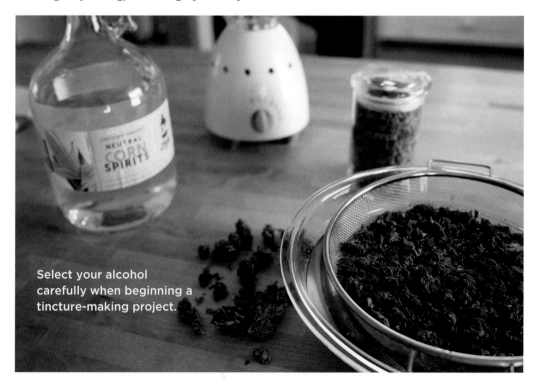

Select your alcohol carefully when beginning a tincture-making project.

THE HERB

Tinctures made with different varieties of marijuana have varying effects because of the entourage effects that the terpenes create. Plant parts being used, maturity at harvest, and post-harvest processing all play a part in determining the tincture's potency. Leaf, trim, bud, kief, and hash are some of the choices, and all are used.

When used for medicinal purposes, a tincture with CBD as well as THC may be beneficial. Some medical tincture makers have adopted cold-processing methods to avoid decarboxylating the cannabinoid acids. Not converting THCa to THC increases possible dosage levels because the THCa does not activate the high, but its medical qualities remain.

If marijuana has been dried and cured as it would be for smoking, some decarboxylation will have already taken place, so THC and CBD will be present without using heat, just not as much. Raw fresh or dried marijuana leaves can be used to make tinctures, though the resulting product may have a chlorophyll flavor. Gently soaking the dried marijuana in water removes some of the chlorophyll, which dissolves in water. Adding a bit of honey to the finished tincture can make it more palatable.

If using fresh plant material, fill a glass container with herb, then add alcohol (ethanol) to the top. If using powdered, dried herb, figure roughly one ounce of weed for every four ounces of alcohol. Use a butter knife to stir the mixture to release air bubbles trapped in the plant material. Cover it. Let it steep in a cool, dark space for two weeks or more. Shake the container daily to mix the ingredients and help the alcohol dissolve the terpenes and cannabinoids. Then strain out the plant material using a sieve lined with cheesecloth set on a glass or metal bowl. The length of time it steeps results in slightly different tinctures. A longer soak extracts more cannabinoids and essential oils, making it stronger and more concentrated, but it also leaches out more of the plant's other chemicals, such as chlorophyll. Splitting a batch between several jars that can be left to steep for differing amounts of time can help you determine what works best for you.

If you're using dried marijuana and want a tincture with the most punch possible, carefully heat the marijuana first. Just spread the

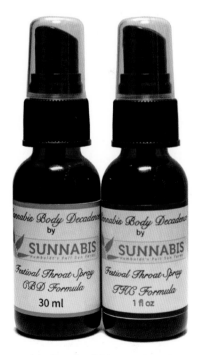

Sunnabis Festival Throat Spray uses carefully selected strains high in CBD and THC, that create a lubricating throat spray designed to maintain your voice at events.

leaves, trim, or bud on a cookie sheet and put it in the oven at 125°F (52°C) for an hour. This decarboxylates the THCA and other cannabinoid acids to a more potent form. Heating at a higher temperature would cause most of the terpenes to evaporate. Higher temperatures also convert THC to the less potent, more sedative CBN. There is no need to grind the marijuana before adding it to alcohol because the cannabinoids and terpenes are almost all on the surface. Grinding results in more sludge collecting at the bottom.

When the same material is used repeatedly to extract cold-water hash, each pull will have a lower quality, with more vegetative material and a strong botanical smell, but it is excellent for making tinctures. Be sure to filter the collected material using screens, high-grade cheesecloth, or a coffee filter.

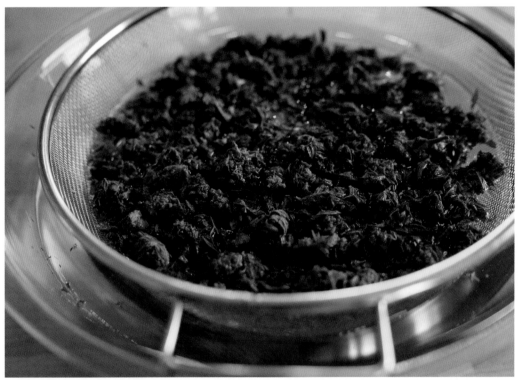

Straining bud with a colander.

STRAINING

To strain the tincture, line a sieve or metal colander with cheesecloth and place it over a clean metal or glass bowl. Pick the type of cheesecloth based on how big the plant particles are that you want to catch. Cheesecloth comes in different grades, based on how tight the weave is, just as printing screens that can be used for sifting kief are graded based on how fine the mesh is. Cheesecloth grades range from the very loosely woven #10 to the extra-fine #90. Unlike the symmetrical mesh of metal and plastic sifting screens, the number of threads per inch in cheesecloth varies horizontally and vertically, as seen below.

Use a looser grade for straining freshly chopped plant material; it catches the plant material and does not clog. Cheesecloth grade #60 to grade #90 is best for straining ground and powdered dried herb for tincture making to avoid sludge build-up. Using fine-grade cloth requires patience because it takes a long time for the extract to seep through. Once gravity has done all it can to pull the tincture through, lift the cheesecloth carefully up by the corners from the sieve and squeeze any remaining solution into the bowl.

If kief or powdered, dry herb is used to make tincture, even the finest cheesecloth or pastry cloth will let some sludge particles through. A second pass through a paper coffee filter or a #1 laboratory filter yields a cleaner, particulate-free product.

Another way to separate the dissolved THC and terpenes from the brew is to use a colander lined with cheesecloth to remove most of the particles. Squeeze the solution from the cloth. Place the cloth back in a bowl and add virgin alcohol. Dip the bag as if it were a teabag to capture more cannabinoids in the alcohol. Warming it gently on a well-ventilated electric stove to about 100°F (38°C) makes the cannabinoids more soluble. Careful: Alcohol fumes are explosive so this should be done in a well-ventilated space or outdoors. Add the new cannabinoid solution to the first one.

Place the solution in a wide-mouth glass jar or pitcher and cover it. Then let it sit in a cool dark place undisturbed for several days or more. Vegetative material mixed into the liquid will separate, either floating to the top or sinking to the bottom. The alcohol solution is fairly pure. Gently skim the floating material from the top. Then siphon the solution from the top, leaving the sunken particulates undisturbed. The siphoned solution can easily be purified further using fine filters, which it passes through very quickly.

ASK ED'S FAST-TRACK TINCTURE

Traditional tincture recipes talk about an aging process: "Let the mixture sit for…" The reason that the tincture gets stronger as it ages is that, at least in theory, more of the THC and other cannabinoids dissolve in the alcohol as time passes. This method speeds up the process by giving the dissolving cannabinoids a quick mechanical assist.

Equipment
  Disposable neoprene or latex gloves
  Blender
  Metal slotted serving spoon
  Colander
  Fine mesh strainer
  Glass or stainless steel bowl, sized to hold colander
  Cloth kitchen towel

Amber or cobalt blue glass jar with sealing lid

Funnel (optional)

Ingredients

Bud, trim, or leaf material

Grain neutral spirits such as Everclear or overproof alcohol such as 151 rum or vodka

Method

1. Weigh the marijuana. For every ounce of herb use ten fluid ounces of alcohol. A 750 ml bottle of alcohol is 25.4 fluid ounces, so a full bottle is good for just over two and a half ounces of weed. Don't forget to decarboxylate the material prior to beginning this process.

2. Place the marijuana in a colander up to one-third full. Do not break up the leaves or buds so that the glands remain on the leaf surfaces. Place the marijuana-filled colander in a mixing bowl. Add enough cool—not cold—water so that the marijuana can spread out. Let the weed sit in the water bath for an hour or so to dissolve the nonactive, water-soluble pigments and carbohydrates from the plant material.

3. Pull the colander from the water and let the water strain out of the plant material. Wearing gloves, roll the marijuana into a ball. Wrap it in a clean dish towel and squeeze out as much water as possible.

4. Place the strained plant material in a blender. Add ten ounces of alcohol for each ounce of marijuana. Place the cover on the blender. Blend at the lowest setting for five minutes. Let it sit for an hour, and then blend on low again for five minutes. Pour the blend into a bowl or wide mouth pitcher. Let the mixture sit for a couple of hours so that the leaf floats to the top of the alcohol.

5. Using a slotted spoon, remove the large floating debris and put it in the fine mesh strainer with the mixing bowl underneath to catch the drainage. Using gloves, press the herb against the strainer to squeeze out the liquid into the bowl. Break up the ball and let it soak in a small amount of virgin alcohol to dissolve remaining cannabinoids. Then repeat the squeezing process, and discard the plant material. It can also be used as a poultice.

6. Pour the liquid through the fine mesh strainer over the bowl. Depending on how fine the mesh and how good the blender, you may see tiny insoluble plant particles in the bowl. If so, filter the tincture through a coffee filter or ultra-fine cheesecloth. If you are using a funnel for transferring the tincture to jars for storage, put the coffee filter or fine cheesecloth inside the funnel and filter while you fill. The tincture is ready to use but a little raw.

7. Test the tincture. Ideally a dose will be no less than a dropper full. If it is too strong,

add alcohol or water. If it is not strong enough, concentrate it by evaporating some of the alcohol. Placing the marijuana in an open mixing bowl in a warm room speeds alcohol evaporation. Covering the bowl or jar with cheesecloth slows evaporation but keeps out dust and dander. Within a few hours the bowl will contain visibly less liquid. Once the tincture is concentrated to the strength desired, put it in a clean, dark glass container and seal it tightly. Store refrigerated in the dark. Long exposure to warmth and oxygen degrades cannabinoid content.

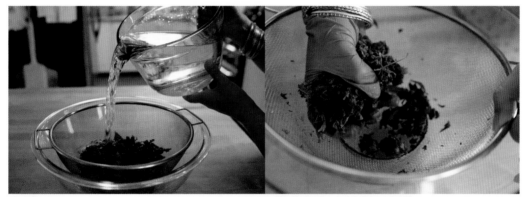

Strain **Roll material into a ball**

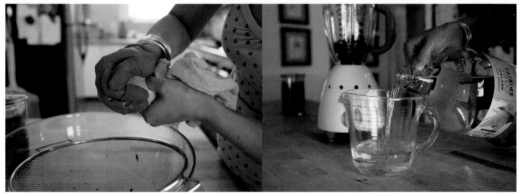

Wring out material with a clean dish towel **Measure alcohol**

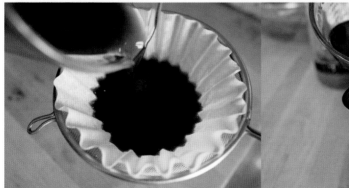
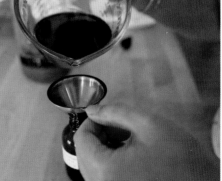

Pour the liquid though a strainer or filter **Bottle the tincture** Photos by Lizzie Fritz

BOTTLING AND STORAGE

Once you've filtered the tincture, use a funnel to fill the storage bottles. Tincture bottles, sometimes called "Boston rounds," should be glass and either amber (brown) or cobalt blue. Do not use clear glass—light causes the cannabinoids to degrade. Do not use plastic bottles—the alcohol will leach potentially harmful chemicals from the plastic. Amber glass bottles are widely available in sizes from 0.5 ounces to 32 ounces. The most common sizes for use with droppers are between 0.5 and 4 ounces.

For applying the tincture, you will want at least one or two tops with built-in droppers sized to the depth of the bottle. For storage, use regular, solid screw caps; they seal better.

Label the tinctures by variety, solute, and date. Keep tinctures in a refrigerator, which slows degradation of cannabinoids to a crawl. They can be stored for years, without losing much potency.

REDUCING TINCTURES TO OIL AND DISTILLATES

Cannabinoid-rich oil can easily be extracted from alcohol tinctures because alcohol evaporates rapidly, particularly when heat is applied.

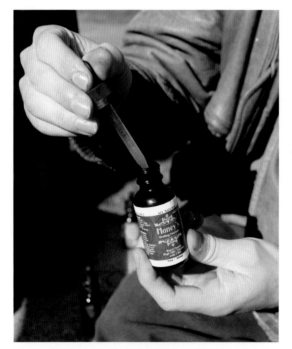

Honey's Healing Royal Purple THC-rich tincture with a sweet glycerin base are good for relaxation, pain management and promoting calm.

A SLOW BUT SAFE NO-EFFORT METHOD

Alcohol evaporates at room temperature, so leaving the top off the tincture bottle or putting the tincture in a bowl or pan for a while reduces it. This works, but it is slower. Remember to cover the jar, bowl, or pan with fine-grade cheesecloth to keep out dust and dander.

THE FASTER HEAT METHOD

Alcohol boils at 173°F (78°C), below the temperature at which cannabinoids vaporize. That means careful use of controlled heat can be used to boil off alcohol from a tincture, leaving only cannabis oil.

Remember: Alcohol is highly flammable—its fumes are explosive. Use a double boiler over an electric hot plate (no flame) to evaporate the alcohol. Provide ventilation, removing the fumes from the space, or work in an open outdoor space.

Rules for Heating Alcohol
- Avoid open flames.
- Don't use gas stoves or pilot lights.
- Use only electric stoves that have a protected heating section.
- Absolutely no smoking or vaporizing anywhere in the vicinity.
- Work in an extremely well-ventilated area—preferably with a lab ventilator.
- Keep windows open and ventilated using box fans turned to blow air out of the room.
- Wear cotton clothing. Do not wear wool or silk, which produce sparks of static electricity.

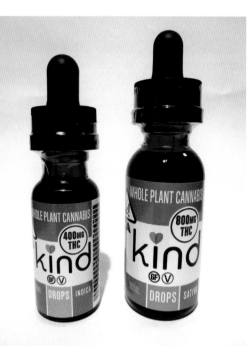

Tinctures can be made from Indica, Sativa or CBD strains like Kind Drops by Kind Medicine which uses whole-plant cannabis infused in olive oil.

Temperature control is critical when reducing tinctures. Never heat a tincture by placing it directly on a burner or stove top, as there will be large differences between the temperature at the bottom and the top. The overheated bottom will produce chemical changes in the extracted oil that will rob it of potent cannabinoids.

Use a double boiler to heat the tincture with less worry. It heats more evenly and the temperature won't exceed 212°F (100°C), the boiling temperature of water. To maintain a lower temperature, use a candy thermometer to check the water in the bottom of the double boiler, or the tincture in the top part. While reducing, stir the tincture frequently with a long spoon or metal kebob skewer.

You can tell when the alcohol has all boiled off because the small alcohol bubbles disappear, leaving the purified oil. The telltale alcohol smell will also disappear.

A basting syringe works well for pulling the oil out of the double boiler. If the oil has particulate matter in it, filter it again through a coffee or lab filter.

This method can also be used to increase the strength of an alcohol tincture without reducing it all the way to oil. Just pull the tincture once the volume has been reduced to the level desired. If you've reduced the volume by half, the resulting tincture will be more than twice as strong as what you started with.

Coldfinger Extractor, by Eden Labs, allows for steam distilling terpenes, cryo and warm extraction and solvent recovery in high quantities, at an efficient rate.

DISTILLING

Most distilling equipment used with herbs are glass Soxhlet extractors, named for a German agricultural chemist who invented the design in 1879 to separate lipids (such as cannabinoids) from a solid base substance (such as marijuana). Soxhlet extractors use a basket to hold the plant material as heated alcohol or other liquid solvent condenses and drips into it. The warm solvent pulls the oils from the plant material and empties into a siphon arm that returns the oil-laden solvent to the distillation flask, where it is reheated and the process of vaporizing and condensing repeats. This is the same principle that is used in percolator-type coffee pots.

As product demand increases, more sizeable and advanced methodologies such as vacuum or pressure-assisted alcohol extraction or centrifugal alcohol extraction have been implemented to Improve the scale of the processing industry. These processes involve manipulating the properties (i.e. temperature, pressure, agitation) of the alcohol to extract higher-purity and/or quality extracts and oils. Larger-scale operations may use increased agitation and/or heat to extract more content from the plant for further separation in post processing. Utilizing a plant material loading vessel, ideally made of glass or stainless steel for chemical inertness, one may load biomass into the vessel, and pour/soak clean alcohol solvent over the material. If desired, the user may choose to manipulate the solvent's temperature to alter selectivity for different types of extracts.

From here, the alcohol may be evacuated from the vessel via vacuum pressure and then fed into a solvent recovery device, such as a rotary evaporator, benchtop still, or similar. Devices like a rotary evaporator utilize heat, agitation, and vacuum to lower the boiling point of constituents to allow for low-temperature and efficient solvent recovery. The recovered solvent may then be reused for extraction, purification, etc. The residual oil may then be emptied from the rotary evaporator, further purged In a vacuum oven (for smoking/vaporization) to remove residual solvent or decarboxylated (activated via heat) if to be used for consumption or in preparation for cannabinoid distillation.

Cannabinoid distillation, specifically Short Path Distillation has become a widely used and accepted method of purifying cannabis oils into a high-clarity, high-potency, fully activated concentrates. Companies such as Lab Society (Colorado) offer various distillation systems that utilize high-vacuum, temperature, and agitation to separate non-cannabinoid compounds present in cannabis extracts/oils away from cannabinoids to achieve high potency (90-99% cannabinoid potencies) distillates. Cannabinoid distillate is typically rendered odorless and tasteless (if done properly) and can help to remove contaminants. It should be noted that this process does not remove all contaminants, specifically fat/oil-soluble pesticides with higher boiling points; other methodologies utilized in conjunction with this process instructed by Elevated Research Solutions (ERS) may be utilized for pesticide removal. Lab Society/ERS is a laboratory equipment and consulting company based out of Colorado, they offer just about any scientific/laboratory equipment, training courses, and consulting services. Utilizing high-potency, odorless, tasteless, and fully-activated concentrates is extremely beneficial for product development as it eases product development, increases end product quality, and Increases product consistency. Other sectors of the market and current medical science, require full spectrum, whole plant products for utilization of The Entourage Effect and health of the Endocannabinoid system.

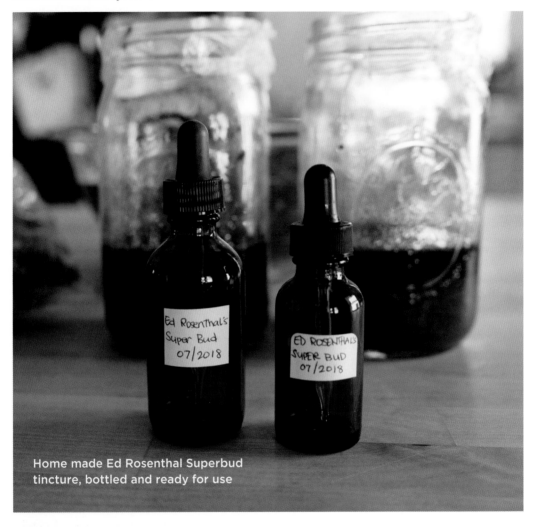

Home made Ed Rosenthal Superbud tincture, bottled and ready for use

GLYCERIN TINCTURES

Alcohol is the standard for making tinctures and it has the advantage of being a great preservative, but for people who cannot tolerate even a drop of alcohol, glycerin tinctures offer an alternative. Some tincture makers use a combination of alcohol and glycerin in their products. Glycerin tinctures are available at many dispensaries, but making your own is not much more involved than making an alcohol tincture. It takes just a few extra steps.

If you have a pure cannabis oil extract, you can make a glycerin tincture by adding a judicious amount of the oil to a bottle of glycerin. Warming it gently (but not too much) and stirring or shaking helps it mix. Pure USP-grade glycerin is inexpensive and available at drug stores everywhere and online.

If making a glycerin tincture from scratch, start by making a carefully strained alcohol tincture. Once you have that, add the alcohol tincture to a comparable amount of glycerin, then evaporate the alcohol. The potency of the glycerin tincture can be adjusted by using either more or less glycerin than the volume of alcohol in the tincture.

One easy method of evaporating the alcohol from the glycerin is to heat it in a double boiler. Measure out the alcohol tincture. To maintain the same strength, add slightly less glycerin, because some of the tincture volume is the cannabis oil. Pour in the alcohol tincture. Using a spoon or spatula, blend them. The larger the surface area of the mixture relative to its depth, the faster alcohol evaporates, so keep the mix limited to a few inches of depth. You'll know when the process is complete because the pan will no longer emit the telltale smell of alcohol. Glycerin tinctures spoil in a few weeks if not refrigerated.

Starting with an alcohol tincture may seem like an unnecessary step, as it is possible to make glycerin tinctures directly. But alcohol is much more efficient at extracting the cannabinoids and other essential oils from marijuana.

You may encounter people who say you can use your oven to evaporate the alcohol from a tincture, either to make a glycerin tincture or to reduce it to oil. Don't do it. The flash point of pure ethyl alcohol vapor is only about 80°F (27°C), and it only takes 3.3% alcohol vapor volume to produce an explosion. Electric ovens may let you get away with more, but even pot roasts braised in a few cups of wine have been known to end with a bang. Using a double boiler in a well-ventilated area or outdoors is a safe way to evaporate alcohol.

THE EFFECTS AND EFFECTIVENESS OF TINCTURE

Tinctures are administered by dropper under the tongue, or sublingually. Th cannabinoids are absorbed by the mucous membranes under the tongue and elsewhere in the mouth and upper throat, releasing them into the bloodstream. Most do not pass through the digestive system, though some can, particularly larger doses, but go directly into the bloodstream. Inhaled cannabis vapor or smoke passes into the bloodstream in the lungs. Direct absorption is an advantage for several reasons: it takes much less time than digestion—it's almost as fast as inhaling, it's easy to titrate because the effects come on rapidly, and the effects are similar to inhaling rather than ingesting.

When substances pass through the digestive system, it takes a minimum of 25 minutes to start feeling their effects, and 45 minutes to an hour before they peak. When there is food in your stomach it takes longer. Swallowed cannabis products pass through the liver which filters what passes into the bloodstream, including some of the cannabinoids. Some of them never reach your bloodstream or your brain. Those cannabinoids that do make it through are subject to the digestive process, which alters THC, so its effects differ from cannabinoids going directly into the bloodstream.

Figuring out tincture dose is much easier than with edibles. The onset of effects is still not nearly as fast as inhalation—which is felt in a matter of seconds—but five minutes after taking the tincture, you can adjust titration. Full effects are felt about 20 minutes after dosage.

Historically, the variable potency of cannabis plants used to make tinctures hindered their use as a modern medicine and contributed to the removal of cannabis from the United States Pharmacopeia. Those two teaspoons that did the trick with one bottle might not in the next batch, making it hard for doctors to prescribe doses with confidence. No one knew what chemicals were in the plant. For the home or artisanal tincture maker, consistency is now less of a challenge. When prepared in one batch or in many small batches from the same plant material, the modern tincture maker has a much easier time creating consistent doses than turn-of-the-century pharmaceutical companies did.

Some people say that tinctures don't affect them much or don't produce the full spectrum of desired effects. Odds are, these people just haven't run across a tincture made properly from cannabis worth extracting. A well-made extract is both a very pleasant and effective way to administer cannabinoids without smoking. It is an excellent choice in no smoking/no vaping situations. You can use cannabis unobtrusively almost anywhere, whether in a theater, traveling or in a park.

ADVANTAGES TO TINCTURES

- Cannabis tinctures deliver the effects of smoking with just a short delay. Since they are not burned, no tars or other pyrolytic compounds are inhaled.
- Tinctures are very discreet. The bottle looks like a regular over-the-counter homeopathic medicine. There is no telltale smell to notice as you self-titrate. There is no need to sneak around.
- The Proper Dose: Once you have used a particular batch a few times, you will figure out the right dose. Tinctures differ as a result of the cannabinoids and, just as importantly, the terpenes that are present. Plant profiles are part of the equation and processing is the other.
- Tolerance to tinctures differs, just as their tolerance to smoked products varies. Start with small doses, adjusting upward as necessary after waiting at least 45 minutes to gauge effects. Tincture doses typically range between the contents of one dropper (approximately 30–40 drops) and six droppers, but some tinctures are much more potent. Since both tincture potency and people's tolerances differ, there is no way to prescribe a dose without knowing the person and the particular tincture.

STORAGE

Label bottles with the date and tincture information to differentiate batches. Tinctures stay potent indefinitely when kept in a cool dark environment, as compared with glycerine-based tinctures that spoil eventually if not kept refrigerated. The main dangers to a tincture's integrity are heat, light, and oxygen. The best storage for a tincture is in a dark-colored glass container that is sealed and kept in a refrigerator or freezer.

MULTIHERBAL TINCTURE

If medicinal applications are your interest, then combining a cannabis tincture with other herbs or herbal extracts may be worth experimentation.

Many other herbs can be used with marijuana to create a synergistic effect. Valerian root, passion flower, lemon balm, and marjoram are calming, reduce anxiety, and aid in sleep. Clove extract can be combined with marijuana tincture for an herbal toothache remedy that is rubbed on the gums.

Additional research into herbal combinations is recommended. Consulting an herbalist may yield a multitude of interesting, personalized extracts.

TYPES OF ALCOHOL

Know the difference between ethanol alcohol versus denatured and isopropyl alcohol. Ethanol-based tinctures and extracts can be ingested or used topically. Extracts made with isopropyl alcohol are poisonous and cannot be ingested safely. They can only be used externally.

Ethanol is sometimes called ethyl alcohol. If buying medical or laboratory-grade ethanol, double check to be sure that it has not been denatured. Denatured ethanol is the kind put in vehicles.

Denatured ethanol and isopropyl are poisonous taken internally and can kill you. They can be used to make topical products for external use only. They should never be consumed or ingested.

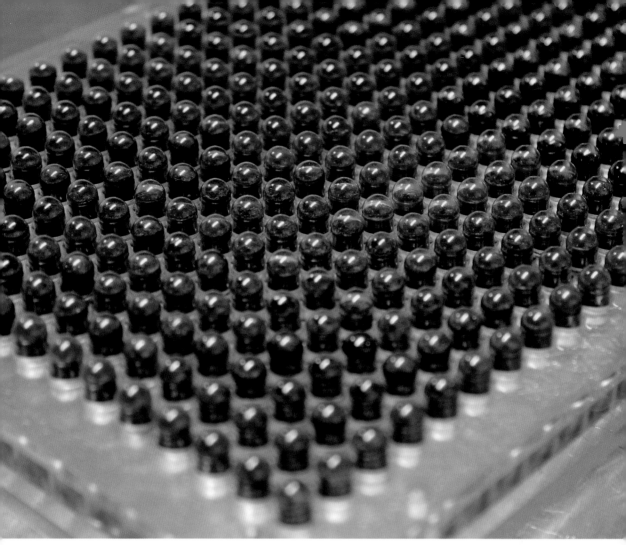

Capsules that have just been filled by hand at Kind Medicine's facility near Santa Cruz, CA.

CAPSULES

We've all been in situations where it's just not cool to smoke. Maybe you've wondered if it's possible to take a marijuana pill. Popping a pill in your mouth with a gulp of water to enjoy the therapeutic and mind-enhancing effects of cannabis would sure be easier and more discrete than firing up a spleef. Turns out you can. Marijuana capsules, also called "maripills" or "canna caps," are very effective and quite easy to make. What's more, they will produce a longer-lasting and somewhat different high than smoking or vaping.

A pill and a pipe won't produce the same effects, even if they contain the same variety and amount of marijuana. The digestive process creates somewhat different metabolites from inhaled marijuana, and those have different effects than the smoked form.

One difference is time: how long it takes to be effective and how long the high will last. Take a puff, and the effects are felt within seconds, letting you easily judge how high you're getting. Take a pill, and you won't know for a while. Anything that gets into your system through your stomach takes much longer to be felt, and that can make knowing how much you have on

board hard to manage. After 15 or 20 minutes of not feeling much effect, it's easy to think you should just go ahead and pop another canna cap or eat another brownie. Then it starts to really hit you just a few minutes later, but by then you've got a lot more coming. For best results, wait at least an hour before upping the dose.

Just as taking a canna cap or edible takes longer to be felt than inhalation, the effects are also extended. The high from smoking a bowl may have mostly worn off after a couple of hours, but the buzz from a brownie or canna cap will just be getting going. Since digestion takes longer than absorbing through your lungs, that hour or more it takes for your stomach to process what you put in it is like an extended-release for THC and the other cannabinoids. That means that the effects will last at least twice as long, depending somewhat on how much you take.

Those longer-lasting effects make oral ingestion just the ticket for many medical marijuana patients who have trouble sleeping without it or need to go longer between doses for other reasons. Some people prefer the high they get from oral marijuana preparations, and those who use it for chronic pain management often say it works better that way. More of a body high and relaxation is how many describe it, but as with all things marijuana, much of the effect has to do with who is using it and what space they are in.

Cannabinated foods are not always predictable. Canna caps are a more consistent and convenient alternative. Marijuana capsules begin to take effect 30–90 minutes after being eaten, depending on whether you take them with food or on an empty stomach. With capsules, it is easier to monitor the exact amount of cannabis that is being ingested. Psychoactive effects typically last 4 to 8 hours, but the herb's medicinal effects infrequently continue for as long as 12 hours.

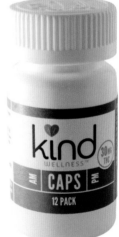

Because canna caps allow cannabis to be eaten without food, these capsules give people more choices. When taken on an empty stomach, the high comes on more quickly, and may be more potent, though some people report eating a light meal within an hour helps enhance the effects. When taken following a meal, assimilation is slower, and the effect is mellower but lasts longer. Medical users may find this increased control over effects beneficial.

The whole cannabis plant is used to make Kind Medicine's Kind Caps inside a gelatin capsule. For anyone with a food allergy, capsules are a simple and effective way to consume cannabis edibles.

CANNA CAPS VERSUS MARINOL

Marinol is the brand name given to dronabinol, which consists of synthetic delta-9 THC suspended in a sesame oil base. This is the only cannabis-based medicine currently legal and available by prescription. It's also very expensive.

Some patients experience good results when using Marinol but others find that it produces anxiety or makes them unpleasantly high because it is only the most psychoactive cannabinoid and it lacks cannabidiol (CBD), which counteracts the anxiety-inducing effects of THC.

More importantly for patients seeking the maximum benefit from cannabis, with Marinol you miss out on the "entourage effect" of marijuana's other cannabinoids working together to increase their overall effectiveness. Research has revealed that the aromatic terpenes that give marijuana its distinctive odor make THC three to four times more effective than it is when taken alone. Those other cannabinoids don't just help THC do a better job. They have therapeutic properties of their own, including relieving pain, inflammation, spasm, nausea, and anxiety.

Most modern cannabis contains mostly THC with negligible amounts of other cannabinoids. Some varieties contain CBD, cannabidiol, a nonpsychoactive cannabinoid that has therapeutic properties such as controlling inflammation and anxiety relief. Another cannabinoid, CBG, that is also nonpsychoactive but may have medical effects, is occasionally present.

Since dronabinol does not contain cannabinoids other than THC and does not include terpenes, it is less effective and is more likely to have uncomfortable side effects such as anxiety and paranoia.

Marinol does, of course, have one irrefutable upside—it has passed muster with the Food and Drug Administration and can be prescribed and possessed legally. As a standardized medicine, dosage is exact to a degree that homemade preparations are incapable of matching. Marinol is approved for treating nausea and vomiting resulting from cancer chemotherapy, and for loss of appetite and weight loss related to HIV infection.

Additional cannabis-derived medicines are available by prescription. GW Pharmaceuticals produces Sativex, a dose-controlled plant extract that is half THC, half CBD, in an alcohol-based tincture that is sprayed under the tongue. Sativex is available by prescription for MS and intractable cancer pain in Canada and 23 other countries.

In the meantime, the best option for getting full-spectrum cannabinoids in a discreet and easy-to-use capsule is to make them yourself from quality cannabis. The homemade canna caps discussed in this chapter are made from leaf, trim, or bud, and offer the complete range of therapeutic cannabinoids. Unlike standardized, dosage-controlled pills made by pharmaceutical companies, homemade marijuana capsules will vary in potency from batch to batch, so the dosage should be tested and adjusted each time new capsules are made.

Marijuana capsules can be made either with powdered cannabis or with an oil-based extract. In either case, heat is used to potentiate the THC. Once the material has been processed, it can be packed into gelatin capsules using a large syringe and a small, inexpensive capsule-filling device.

Gelatin capsules and capsule-filling machines are available at many health food stores or online. Capsule-filling machines are small (about the size of a brick) and inexpensive (under

$20). They simply hold the gelatin capsule in place, allowing many pills to be made at one time.

If you are a strict vegetarian, gelatin capsules may not be for you as they are made from cows. Vegetarian capsules made of starch are available, but they are inadvisable for this process, because they dissolve when exposed to oil. Ask a salesperson if the vegetarian capsules they offer can tolerate an oilbased filling before purchasing them for canna cap use.

Size #0 capsules are recommended because their small size is not too difficult to swallow. Size #0 can hold 325 milligrams of marijuana preparation. Dosage may vary between 1 and 5 capsules, depending on the potency of the material used. The largest size most people can tolerate is #00 size. The larger size makes preparing them easier, and both the capsules and machines are widely available from health food stores or online. This size has a capacity of 650 milligrams. Usually 1–2 pills at this size comprise a sufficient dose.

HOW TO MAKE CANNA CAPS

Canna caps can be made from leaf and trim only, bud only, or a leaf/bud combination. No matter what is used, it is necessary to process the plant material before filling capsules. There are three basic ways cannabis can be capsulized: as just dry powder, as powder mixed with an oil, or as an oil extract of the cannabis.

All three methods need the plant material to be heated a bit to "decarboxylate" it, a chemical process that changes the cannabinoids found in the plant—THCa and CBDa, which are non-psychoactive—to the active form by releasing COOH from the molecule. That process happens naturally when you smoke or vaporize marijuana, but for preparations you swallow, it needs to be done separately.

Mild heat, about 100°F (38°C), also helps the cannabinoids bind to the oil, if that's the method you're using. Packing the capsules with a mixture of marijuana and oil makes it easier for the body to digest and utilize the herb. Whole plant material contains not only the bulbous THC-containing glands but also the microscopic—and sharp—hairs on which they rest. Oil and heat soften these spiky hairs, making them less irritating to the stomach.

The cannabinoids and other essential oils that produce marijuana's effects are soluble in fats, oils, and alcohol. They are not soluble in water. Gelatin caps hold nonaqueous liquids such as oil and alcohol, but they dissolve when filled with water. Luckily, marijuana is mixed with these liquids, not water.

Some people find that, even after processing, they have trouble digesting pills that use leaf material. If this is the case, try using hash or kief. Both kief and hash contain much less vegetative matter. The tiny hairs from the vegetative matter are most likely the culprits in digestive complaints.

If that's a problem, just make your canna caps with the strained oil method described below.

Equipment and Ingredients
- Cooking oil (coconut, olive, or canola)
- Plant material (bud, leaf, trim, or a combination)
- Food processor or flour mill (when leaf/trim is used)
- Clean or unused coffee grinder
- Flour sifter (optional)
- Crockpot, double boiler, or small saucepan
- Candy thermometer (optional)
- Gelatin capsules
- Capsule-filling machine
- Tamping tool if using vegetative material (machine may come with one; otherwise, the head of a nail works well)
- Large syringe (if using oil only)
- Paper cone coffee filter (if using oil only)
- Cookie sheet

PROCESSING LEAF AND BUD FOR CAPSULES

Clean the leaf, trim, or cured bud carefully before starting the capsule-making process. Make sure there are no small stems in your material. Kief and hash are already well suited to capsule making, though caution should be used with dosage, as the end product may be very potent.

The material should be very dry before beginning this process. Spread the material on a cookie sheet and place it in an oven at 100°F (38°C) for an hour to remove the last remnants of moisture and decarboxylate it

Chop the material into a fine powder or flour using a coffee grinder or blender. This processing generates clouds of cannabis dust that contain many glands that can be retained by letting the dust settle before you open the top.

If the material contains a lot of leaf, follow the coffee-grinding step with an additional pass through a flour sifter. This last step makes the material finer and more consistent by separating out any large pieces.

Don't skimp on material. It is always better to have more marijuana powder than you plan to use, so if too much oil is added accidentally, a little more powder can also be added to reach the right consistency. Extra capsule powder can be stored in the freezer. The refrigerator is also adequate. Cold, dark, and oxygen-free conditions preserve marijuana's potency and protect it against molds or bacteria.

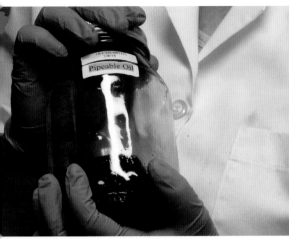

Pipeable cannabis oil ready to put into capsules

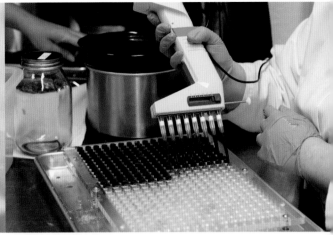

Filling capsules by hand

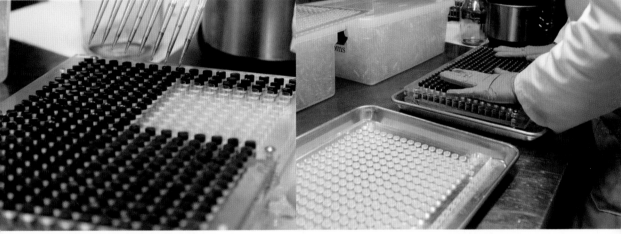

Topping off each capsule for equal-fill levels

Capsule tops are applied with a top applicator board.

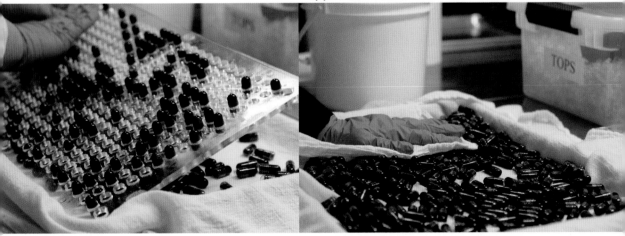

A finished batch of capsules ready for cleaning.

Cleaning the capsules to make them ready for packaging

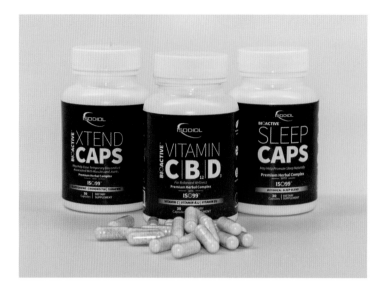

With three formulations for differing uses, Isodiol's Bioactive Caps are made with CBD and other additions like vitamins to promote health.

MAKING THE FILLING

PURE CANNA OIL CAPS

Some of the best canna caps are made with strained coconut oil cannabis preparations. Coconut oil works well because it is a soft solid at room temperature, is readily available in pure organic forms from health food stores, and is almost 100% nonhydrogenated fat, so it's healthful in its own right. Olive oil is another popular medium because it is healthful and stable at room temperature.

To heat the oil and cannabis, a double boiler or Crockpot works well and helps ensure you don't overheat it. As with other marijuana preparations, keeping heat low is key to preserving the cannabinoids that will vaporize and escape when temperatures get above 280°F (138 °C).

CALCULATING QUANTITIES

Capsule machines may make 24, 50, or 100 capsules at a time. Size #0 capsules hold 0.3 grams, and #00 capsules hold 0.6 grams. The amount it takes to fill 50 capsules is 15 grams (about a half-ounce) for size #0, and 30 grams (about 1 ounce) for #00.

Place the desired amount of oil in a double boiler or Crockpot. A small frying pan or saucepan will also work if care is taken to keep the temperature at 100°F (38°C). (That's where the candy thermometer comes in.) Once the oil has warmed, add the ground marijuana, stirring to coat the material thoroughly.

If you are straining out the plant material to make oil-only capsules, the longer you let the mixture heat, the better. It takes a while for all of the cannabinoids and plant oils to bind to the coconut oil. Half an hour is the minimum, an hour captures almost all the THC, and six hours is great for the obsessive. Using a Crockpot or other slow cooker saves you constantly monitoring the heat. The oil-to-powder ratio varies between 3–8 tablespoons per ounce because leaf and bud absorb oil in different quantities. Use just enough oil to make the material stick together in a dry paste-like consistency, particularly if you are using an oil other than coconut that is fluid at room temperature. Too much oil makes filling the capsules more difficult. More powder should be added if the mixture seems too oily.

The mixture should keep the same dark green color it started with. If the material turns brown, it has burned, which is unfortunate. This material has lost most of its value. You should start over rather than continuing with this material.

If you are using a saucepan or skillet and want capsules that contain all the plant material, heat the oil using a candy thermometer to monitor the exact temperature. Once the temperature reaches 100°F (38°C), remove the pan from the stove and add the plant material to reach the proper consistency. The mixture can be encapsulated when it has cooled to room temperature (below 90°F [32°C]).

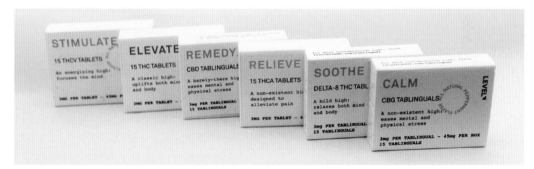

Tablinguals from LEVEL dissolve fully in your mouth and have sublingual effects, as opposed to capsules which are eaten and processed through the liver via an edible. 3mg each make them great for micro-dosing.

FILLING THE CAPSULES

Capsule machines have a platform with holes. The bottom of the capsule shells fit into this platform. The process for filling the capsules is only slightly different for using just the oil or the full plant-oil mix.

For oil-only capsules, heat the mix until it is liquid rather than viscous, fill a large syringe or baster with the oil, then inject it into the capsules one by one. Don't let the mixture get too cool before filling the capsules, or getting it into them will be difficult if not impossible. If it does harden, just gently reheat it to the point of turning to liquid.

For capsules that use the full oil-plant mix, use a spreading card to distribute the oil mixture over the capsule- filling device. Tamp the mixture down into the capsules. Repeat the process until they are completely filled. If your capsule-making kit did not come with a tamper, sterilize a nail with the right-sized head and use it.

STORAGE

Keep canna caps in a sealed, dark glass bottle or jar. They have a shelf life of only a few weeks at room temperature, but in the refrigerator, they keep for months. They can also be stored long term in a freezer.

CAPSULE-MAKING TIPS

- Gelatin caps are derived from animal products. Vegetarian capsules can be used, but some types dissolve when oil is used in the filling. Before buying vegetarian capsules, ask the salesperson if they can be filled with an oil-based mixture.
- It is a good idea to process a little extra powdered material. Then the material-to-oil ratio can be adjusted if too much oil is accidentally mixed in.
- When heating plant material for the capsules, heat it in a double boiler rather than on a stove top to assure keeping a low temperature. THC starts to vaporize at just over 280°F (138 °C). Some terpenes are volatile at 70°F (21°C). If using a burner set it at a very low temperature to avoid ruining the plant material's psychoactive and therapeutic properties. A Crockpot or other slow cooker set on low works well.
- Bud absorbs more oil than leaf material. The amount of oil needed may depend on the ratio of leaf to bud, the type of oil used, and how dry the plant material is.
- Marijuana varieties differ in potency and cannabinoid content. Different strains produce different highs and medicinal qualities. Likewise, using different ratios of trim, bud, leaf, or kief affects potency. Reassess dosage when a new combination of plant material is used.

Using Kief

Kief offers a cleaner alternative to powdered leaf or bud especially for those who find plant material hard to digest. Kief dissolves easily when mixed in warm oil. It does not have a dark green color when mixed and heated because it doesn't contain plant matter. Kief is more concentrated than bud so a kief-packed pill will be more potent. Try size #0 capsules when using kief because the dosing size is smaller.

Doseage

As with all marijuana products, the right dosage depends on the potency of the herb, how you prepare it, and the person taking it. Dosage varies from person to person and from batch to batch, but it usually ranges between one to five size #0 capsules or one to two #00 capsules.

When capsules are made using only powdered bud, they are more potent than a bud/ leaf or leaf/trim mixture. Likewise, kief, which is a concentrated form of marijuana, has a higher potency, and the dosage should be lowered.

Canna caps can be taken at any time, but just like marijuana foods, results depend in part on whether they are eaten on an empty or full stomach. When taken on an empty stomach, the onset of effects is more rapid, and the high may be more intense. Eating food right after the pills are taken may mitigate the potency and delivery, though some say a light meal within an hour enhances the high. If canna caps are taken after a meal, the effects will come on more slowly and the high may be milder. As always, effects will also differ from person to person, so start with small amounts and give it at least 90 minutes to take effect.

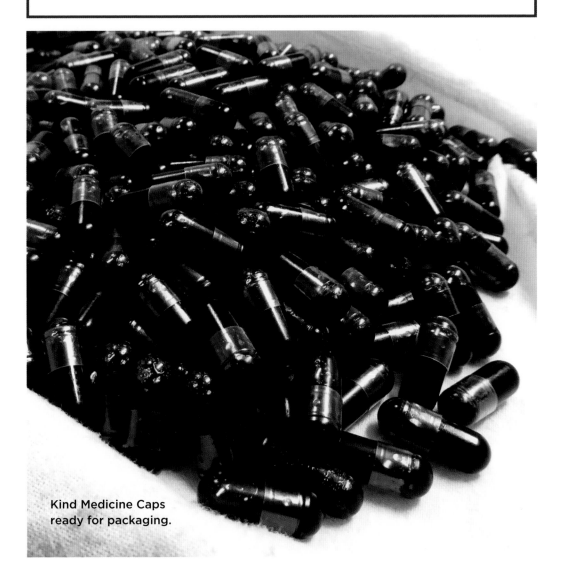

Kind Medicine Caps ready for packaging.

Mary's Medicinals

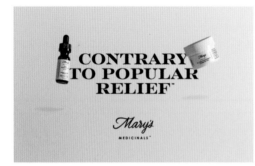

Mary's Medicinals had a simple mission in mind when its founders started the company in 2013: help patients, transform how consumers view and use cannabis, and convert naysayers and skeptics into advocates. Judging from the company's accomplishments thus far, the plan seems to be working.

Headquarted in Denver, Mary's has more than 35 full-time employees, and has a product presence in 11 states where adult recreational and/or medical cannabis use has been legalized. Since its inception, the company's work has been acknowledged with a number of awards, including 2014 Invention of the Year in the Cannabis Business Awards, Most Innovative Product at the CannAwards and Best New Product at the High Times Cannabis Cup.

From the beginning, Mary's founders saw a need for accurately-dosed products and clean delivery methods for those seeking alternatives to smoking cannabis and the psychedelic culture associated with the industry. The company has always recognized the power of the plant beyond its CBD and THC, and has also emphasized the therapeutic possibilities with THCa, CBN and CBC.

Best known for its transdermal applications, Mary's developed a patented transdermal gel that utilizes a proprietary carrier agent to deliver the cannabinoids directly into the bloodstream for rapid relief. The pen dispenses exactly 2mg per pump for 2-3 hours of relief. Mary's also produces patches that are dosed at 10mg and 20mg and provide 8-10 hours of relief. There's a wide array of benefits of transdermal and topical applications such as the elimination of smoking, bypassing first-pass metabolism (from oral administration), dose control, continued release, convenience, ease of use and beneficial systemic effects.

Mary's believes in the benefits of proactive cannabinoid therapy, so most of its products are developed for daily use. The cannabinoids used in its topicals (CBD, CBN, THC, CBC, THCa) and natural terpenes are widely reported to provide pain relief and reduce inflammation. These cannabinoids have also been reported to provide relief for those suffering from psoriasis, dermatitis, acne, epilepsy, Crohn's disease and skin cancers.

When cannabis is administered, cannabinoids bind to receptor sites in the brain and body, and have different effects based on which receptors they bind to and their interaction with that receptor. For example, CBN (Cannabinol) binds with CB-2 receptors located throughout the body, which may explain why patients report that it is a powerful analgesic. With an increasing understanding of the effects of cannabinoids, patients can tailor their cannabinoid consumption to the type of relief they need.

From product research and development to its educational materials, everything Mary's does is to advance the global understanding, acceptance, and adoption of cannabis and other plant-based medicines. The company is committed to the scientific development of products that utilize the endocannabinoid system for human health and will continue to contribute to furthering the understanding of this system.

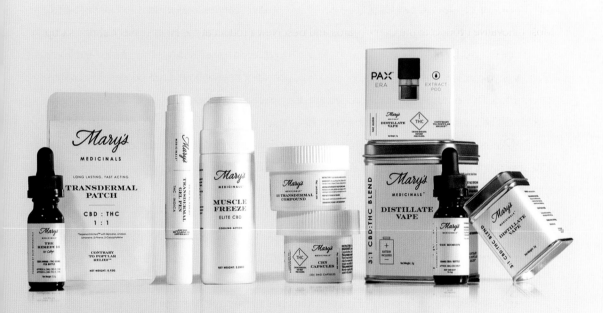

Cannariginals

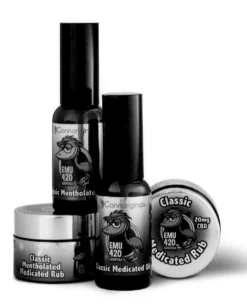

After 20 years in the financial services industry, Gary and Vickie Lowe decided it was time to make a change. Knowing that they wanted to make an impact in the medicinal cannabis industry, they focused in on CBD but weren't satisfied with the delivery mechanisms that were available.

When they set out to design a delivery system for maximum bioavailability, they began experimenting with infusions and different ways to bind cannabinoids with various types of essential oils. Since Gary's father was raising Emu in Oklahoma, they knew about Emu oil and its ability to be a superior transdermal agent. Soon enough, they were working on infusions that led to the development of Cannariginals' Emu 420 Essentials.

"We wanted to get into a space where we felt we could really make a difference and experience a deeper sense of gratitude in our work," says Gary. "It did not take long to realize we were on the right path even if it is a bumpy road in this industry."

Founded January 2014, Cannariginals is located in Bakersfield, California, and the company's products are now sold in over 750 Medical Marijuana Collectives throughout the state. Cannariginals won its first major award in February 2014 at the High Times Cannabis Cup.

Cannariginals produces a number of different products that feature a full transdermal carrier, and capitalize on the natural synergy between Emu oil and cannabis. Emu oil has been long-used by Australian Aborigines for its healing properties, and in research studies it has been shown to provide anti-inflammatory, anti-aging and moisturizing properties. It has an abundance of omega 3-6-9 oils and is hypoallergenic.

In addition to Emu oil, the company's products are created with organic ingredients, and provide a therapeutic punch that goes beyond just the cannabis infusion. Emu oil has an efficient transdermal delivery system and can deeply penetrate the skin's surface faster than many other oils and creams. And because Emu oil does not work its way out of the body quickly, the medicine has a longer lasting effect.

Since starting the company, Gary and Vickie have maintained a strong connection to their community of patients and caregivers, and support causes, events and individuals who are also trying to make a difference. Some of the organizations they support include the Lupus Foundation, Weed4Warriors, and the Epidermolysis Bullosa (EB) Community.

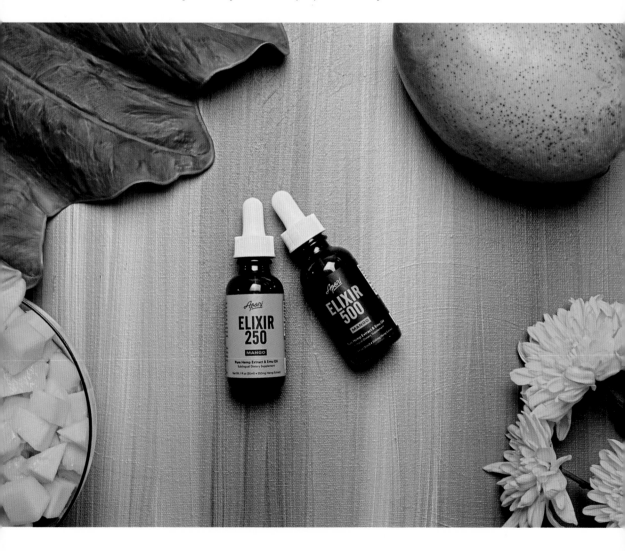

Glossary

Δ-9 Tetrahydrocannabinol: Best known by the abbreviation THC, this is the cannabinoid long thought to be the alpha and omega of cannabis potency, now known to be one of several compounds that contributes to the "entourage effect" (see **Entourage Effect**)

11-Hydroxy-THC: A THC metabolite produced by the human body's metabolization of Δ-9 THC; this iteration of THC metabolizes into the brain more quickly than its precursor, converting to 11-Nor-9-carboxy THC in the process.

11-Nor-9-carboxy THC: Inert secondary metabolite of THC, created by the metabolization of 11-hydroxy-THC; 11-Nor-9-carboxy is the "deactivated" THC remnant that infamously lingers in the body for several months — it is the primary target of urinalysis "drug tests" for cannabis.

710: A numerical signifier for cannabis concentrates — the dab-specific symbolic counterpart to 420; the numbers "spell" the word OIL when read upside-down (also see **Oil**)

Azeotrope: A two-liquid mixture with a constant boiling point; the vapor has the same proportions as the liquid state, making it impossible to separate using distillation (see **Distillation,**

Fractional distillation and **Short path distillation**) necessitating the use of additional solvents to "break" the mixture.

Banger: A small quartz glass or pyrex "bucket" or "trough" attached to a drop stem used for dabbing concentrates (see Dabbing); the contemporary connoisseur standard for low-temp/high flavor dabs.

BHO: Abbreviation for "butane hash oil"; can refer to any number of concentrates derived from butane extraction; also can refer to raw, unpurged, liquid solution of butane and extract bubble hash: cannabis glands concentrated by means of ice water

Cannabinoid: A class of molecules produced by cannabis; there are more than 100 of them. Many interact with the human nervous system to produce the wide variety of cannabis' effects

Carb cap: Small piece of glass fitted to fill the top of a banger, usually with a "carb" hole for airflow; essential tool for taking low-temp dabs, replaced the dome.

CBD: Cannabidiol, the second most common cannabinoid found in cannabis; once an obscurity, now a desirable compound in its own right, highly prized by people seeking the anti-inflammatory and anxiolytic impacts without euphoria or dramatic perceptional shifts.

CBDa: The acidic precursor of CBD; as with THC, the phytocannabinoids (see Phytocannabinoids) produced by the cannabis plant's resin glands are mostly cannabinoid acids, which become THC/CBD respectively through the process of decarboxylation.

Closed loop: An extraction approach that recycles the extraction solvent and contains the process inside a closed system, as opposed to open blasting (see **Open blasting**)

Combustion: The chemical process behind the physical phenomenon known as "burning;" when you smoke a joint, you're combusting the paper and cannabis. This is pleasurable, but it also produces carcinogens and other toxic compounds, which is why some consumers prefer dabbing or vaporization (see **Dabbing** and **Vaporization**)

Conduction: Heat transfer through solid matter, such as metal; a conduction vaporizer has a metal or other hot element as its heat source

Convection: The transfer of heat by automatic circulation of a fluid; a convection vaporizer circulates hot air or fluid to produce the proper temperature

Crystalline: Refers to the molecular structure of a solid; the more orderly that structure is the more it will resemble a crystal. This is the natural state of "pure" cannabinoids, which are solids, and which can be purified and refined using recrystallization processes (see **Recrystallization**)

Dab/Dabbing: Both a noun and a verb; the "dose" of concentrate you vaporize and inhale is known as a dab, as in "I just took a dab of some shatter." You can also say "go ahead and dab some of that shatter," or "I was just dabbing on some shatter." In other words, you can dab a dab and when you do you're dabbing.

Dab rig/Oil rig: A waterpipe specifically designed and fitted for dabbing; different percolators (see Percolators) are used than in a traditional waterpipe and smaller pieces are highly prized, meaning the designs tend to be more stylistically elaborate than classic bongs and pipes.

Decarboxylation: the removal of a carboxyl, which is a carbonate molecule (COOH). When carboxyl molecules are attached to the THC molecule, it is called THCa, or THC acid. In this form, THC lacks most of its psychoactivity. Decarboxylation removes the COOH acid molecule, leaving behind THC. Mild heat is often used to convert THCa to THC. This happens during drying, vaporization, and smoking. Some decarboxylation happens naturally as marijuana cures and ages.

Diamond mining: Also known as "Jar Tech," this is a simple process for recrystallizing freshly extracted BHO; this process works best using live resin (see **Live Resin**)

Distillate: The refined high-cannabinoid extract produced by distilling concentrates; increasingly the most popular option for filling vape pen cartridges (see **Vape pen**)

Distillation: The ancient process of exploiting the discrepancy between respective boiling points for the parts of a mixture to separate and purify them; used in extraction to refine "crude oil"

E-nail: An electrical heating element for a banger or nail (see nail) attached to a temperature controller, allowing for consistent, targeted temperature dabs with no need for a torch; apart from a quick swipe of a Q-tip (see **Q-Tip Tech**) there is no downtime between dabs.

Endocannabinoid: The natural cannabinoids produced in the body by humans and other vertebrate animals that regulate complex biological processes, including those of the immune system; endocannabinoids attach to specific receptors that also respond to phytocannabinoids

Entourage Effect: A phrase coined by foundational cannabis researcher, Dr. Raphael Mechoulam, to describe how multiple compounds present in cannabis (not just THC) are responsible for the plant's clinically confirmed effects.

Fractional distillation: The distillation method used for mixtures with components that have boiling points that are within 25°C of each other, making extraction through simple distillation impossible.

Live resin: BHO produced using live or flash frozen live material; the higher terpene content makes it an ideal choice for producing sauces, sugars and other BHO consistencies that rely on recrystallization.

n-Butane: An organic solvent refined from natural gas; it is the most popular hydrocarbon used in solvent extraction and the chemical cornerstone of the "710" extraction renaissance. It also serves as the fuel for the torch used in dabbing.

Nail: A small, titanium or quartz heating element for vaporizing concentrates; comes with or without a dome

Nucleation: A natural separation process that occurs in all mixtures; in cannabis concentrates this means the separation of the cannabinoid solid from the terpenes, which are natural solvents and fundamentally liquid.

Oil: A catch-all term that refers to any cannabis concentrate produced through solvent extraction, not generally used for hash or rosin.

Open blasting: The original BHO extraction process; filling a tube with weed, blasting butane through the tube and collecting what comes out the other side for purging; not actually as dangerous as often presented, but more or less a non-starter in the current regulatory climate.

Oxidation: The action of oxygen when it unites with another substance chemically. This happens quickly in fire, but also takes place at a much slower pace at room temperature. For marijuana and its products, oxidation is deterioration. The oxygen in air interacts with marijuana to reduce its THC content.

Phase: The state of matter, usually in one of three states: solid, liquid, and gas; supercritical is a fourth state created under unusual conditions

Phytocannabinoids: The cannabinoids produced by plants, as distinguished from endocannabinoids, the ones produced naturally by humans and animals

Purge: The act of removing a solvent from a solution, as occurs during BHO or CO_2 extraction

Pyrolytic compounds: Compounds produced by chemical changes brought about by the action of heat in the absence of oxygen. These compounds often consist of carcinogenic hydrocarbons, often gasses.

Recrystallization: A purification process that stimulates and encourages crystallization of solid components in a mixture.

Resin glands: General term for all trichome types on the cannabis plant (see **trichome)**

Rosin: The refined product of applying heat and pressure to raw buds or hash.

Rosin tech: A mechanical extraction or refinement process for buds an hash respectively; heat and pressure are used to coax a potent, flavorful, full spectrum product that is dabbable.

Shatter: A highly regarded type of BHO characterized by its translucence and its brittleness at room temperature; can range in consistency from "true" brittle shatter (like golden or amber glass) to a sappy Snap n' Pull consistency.

Skillet/Swing: a type of heating element used in dabbing concentrates; direct descendant of hot knifing, immediate predecessor to titanium dome nails.

Solution: When a substance dissolves, its molecules actually form a loose molecular relationship with the liquid that it dissolves into. For instance, sugar in hot water or chlorine in a pool are solutions—their molecules spread out so that they are evenly spaced throughout the liquid.

Solubility: The property of a solid, liquid, or gaseous chemical solute that allows it to dissolve in a solid, liquid, or gaseous solvent to form a homogeneous solution of the solute in the solvent.

Solvent: A substance that dissolves another substance, creating a solution— water is the most basic solvent in the universe; because cannabinoids and terpenes are oils, solvents used to extract them include alcohol, petroleum based liquids and liquid CO_2.

Subcritical: CO_2 extraction done below the critical temperature and pressure point of carbon dioxide when it turns to liquid

Sublimation: A phase change directly from solid to gas without an intermediate liquid phase — the classic example, and the one most relevant to extraction is the sublimation of solid CO_2 or "dry ice" to gaseous carbon dioxide at room temperature.

Sublingual: A method of using tinctures. The liquid is placed and held under the tongue and is absorbed by the porous mucous membranes lining the mouth and throat. When consumed in this way, absorption is faster than eating because it does not pass through the digestive system before entering the bloodstream, but is slower than smoking. This is a good way to use marijuana for the treatment of nausea without inhaling.

Sugar: In this context, refers to "terp sugar," which is a sandy, granular variation of BHO that has a damp appearance and consistency from terpene saturation.

Supercritical: An unusual phase that occurs when a substance is held at or pushed past its critical point when it changes from gas to liquid or similar. A supercritical substance has different characteristics (solubility, diffusivity) than the same substance has as a liquid or a gas; it is considered a "cloud."

Terpene: The volatile aromatic molecules present in plants including cannabis. They are based on a C5 H8 model. They are used in aromatherapy and can affect both mood and physical condition.

Terpene profile: The aroma and flavor identity of a given strain or concentrate; the sum total of all the detectable terpenes.

THCa: The acidic precursor to Δ-9 tetrahydrocannabinol — most of the THC produced by the cannabis plant is actually THCa, which decarboxylates (see **decarboxylation**) to Δ-9 THC when exposed to heat.

Titration: The process of determining the proper dosage for a desired effect

Transdermal: Gradual absorption of a substance through skin contact, often through an adhesive patch; differs from topical in that transdermal applications directly access the bloodstream through the skin, while topical applications only penetrate the skin barrier only minimally, generally to treat the skin itself. Transdermal applications can be perfect for those trying to circumvent gastrointestinal issues.

Vaporization: The act of gently heating cannabis or concentrates to about 380°F (193°C), at which point the THC turns into a gas and can be inhaled without the carcinogens associated with burning the plant

Winterization: In bio-industry, the act of removing waxes from an oil, usually through the application of cold temperature

SOURCES AND ADDITIONAL READING

Note: This book was made possible through generous contributions of knowledge by dozens of cannabis experts; manufacturers that shared their process with us and chemists and lab wizards who helped clarify (and sometimes translate) that information; technological innovators and inventors who showed us the cutting edge of cannabis consumption; the countless cannabis industry professionals who helped make this book a reality. But we also pulled from the broad and ever-expanding body of research and writing around one of the planet's most useful and misunderstood plants — these are all the sources that informed or inspired our writing, even tangentially.

Behavioral Health Services Division. 1983. "The Lynn Pierson Therapeutic Research Program: A Report on Progress to Date." Health and Environment Department: New Mexico.

Board of Pharmacy, State of Tennessee. 1983. "Annual Report: Evaluation of Marijuana and Tetrahydrocannabinol in Treatment of Nausea and/or Vomiting Associated with Cancer Therapy Unresponsive to Conventional Anti-Emetic Therapy: Efficacy and Toxicity".

Brenneisen, Rudolf. (2007). "Chemistry and Analysis of Phytocannabinoids and Other Cannabis Constituents". *Marijuana and the Cannabinoids*. 17-49.

Clayton, G. and F. Clayton, eds., *Patty's Industrial Hygiene and Toxicology*, 3rd rev. ed. New York: Wiley & Sons, 1981.

Connell Clarke, Robert. *Hashish*. Los Angeles, CA: Red Eye Press, 1998.

Earleywine, Mitch and Sara Smucker Barnwell. "Decreased Respiratory Symptoms in Cannabis Users Who Vaporize." *Harm Reduction Journal*, 2007.

ElSohly, M. A., ed. *In Forensic Science and Medicine: Marijuana and the Cannabinoids*. Totowa: NJ: Humana Press, 2007.

Flowers, Tom. *Marijuana Herbal Cookbook*. CA: Flowers Publishing, 1995.

Gieringer, Dale and Scott Goodrich and Joseph St. Laurent. "Cannabis Vaporizer Combines Efficient Delivery of THC with Effective Suppression of Pyrolytic Compounds," in *Journal of Cannabis Therapeutics 4* (1), 2004.

Grotenhermen, Franjo, MD and Ethan Russo, MD, ed. *Cannabis and Cannabinoids: Pharmacology, Toxicology, and Therapeutic Potential*. Binghamton, NY: Hayworth Integrative Healing Press, 2002.

Husnu Can Baser, K. and Gerhard Buchbauer, ed. *Handbook of Essential Oils: Science, Technology, and Applications*. Boca Raton, FL: CRC Press, 2009.

Kemplay, Richard. *Stir Crazy: Cooking with Cannabis*, by Bobcat Press. Oakland, CA: Quick American Archives, 1999.

Iversen, Leslie L. *The Science of Marijuana*. Oxford, UK: Oxford University Press, 2000.

Latta, R. P. and B. J. Eaton. "Seasonal Fluctuations in Cannabinoid Content of Kansas Marijuana." *Economic Botany* 29: 153–163, April–June 1975.

McPartland, J. and E. Russo. "Cannabis and Cannabis Extracts: Greater Than the Sum of Their Parts," *Journal of Cannabis Therapeutics* p.103: 2002.

Mikuriya, Tod H, MD. "Vaporization of Cannabinoids: A Preferable Drug Delivery Route." *Schaffer Library of Drug Policy*, 1993.

Moriarty, Sandy. *Aunt Sandy's Medical Marijuana Cookbook.* Piedmont, CA: Quick American Publishing, 2010.

Pertwee, R. G. "The Diverse CB1 and CB2 Receptor Pharmacology of Three Plant Cannabinoids: Δ9-Tetrahydrocannabinol, Cannabidiol and Δ9-Tetrahydrocannabivarin." *British Journal of Pharmacology* 153 (2): 199–215, January 2008.

Pilcher, Tom. *The Cannabis Cookbook: Over 35 Tasty Recipes for Meals, Munchies, and More.* Philadelphia, PA: Running Press, 2007.

Prentiss, D. et al. "Patterns of Marijuana Use Among Patients With HIV/AIDS Followed in a Public Health Care Setting," *Journal of Acquired Immune Deficiency Syndromes*, 35: 38-45: 2004.

Sicard, Cheri. *The Cannabis Gourmet Cookbook.* Long Beach, CA: Z-Dog Media, 2012.

Sumach, Dr. Alexander. *A Treasury of Hashish.* Toronto, ONT: Stoneworks Publishing Company, 1976.

Upton, Roy, et al, ed. "Standards of Identity, Analysis, and Quality Control." *Cannabis Inflorescence: Cannabis Spp. American Herbal Pharmacopoeia*, 2013.

Werner, Clint. *Marijuana: Gateway to Health.* San Francisco, CA: Dachstar Press, 2011.
"Hash Oil Explosions Increasing Across U.S.," The InfoGram, February 7, 2013.

Williamson, E. "Synergy and Other Interactions in Phytomedicines," *Phytomedicine: International Journal of Phytotherapy and Phytopharmacology* 8: 401-409: 2001.

The U.S. Fire Administration—Emergency Management and Response— Information Sharing and Analysis Center (EMR-ISAC).

MORE STUDIES

CDC Safety Guidelines for Butane
http://www.cdc.gov/niosh/docs/81-123/pdfs/0068.pdf

EPA Butane Exposure Guidelines
http://www.epa.gov/oppt/aegl/pubs/butane_interim_dec_2008_v1.pdf

National Institutes of Health Toxicology Data Network (Butane)
TOXNET.nlm.nih.gov

Praxair Material Safety Data Sheet—Butane
http://www.praxair.com/~/media/North%20America/US/Documents/SDS/ Butane%20C4H10%20 Safety%20Data%20Sheet%20SDS%20P4572.ashx

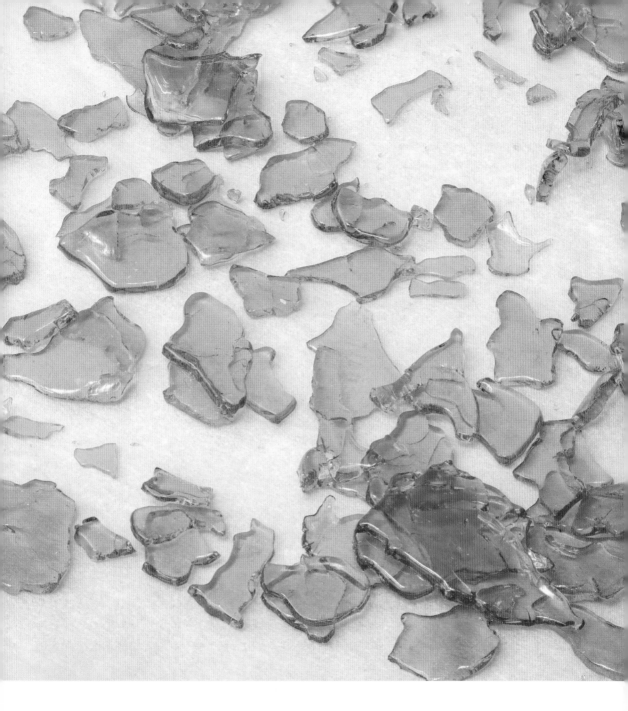

Sponsors

We would like to thank our sponsors, whose support and participation helped make this book possible.

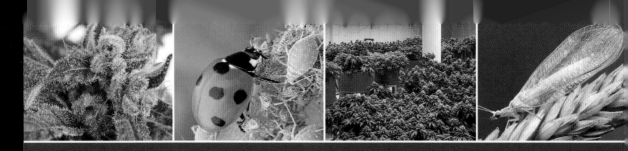

Your #1 Source For Organic Growing Solutions

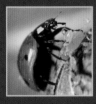

Biological Pest Controls
Beneficial Insects
Beneficial Nematodes
Microorganisms
Predatory Mites

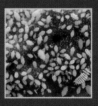

Natural Pesticides
Biorational Insecticides
Mycoinsecticides
Miticides
Traps & Lures

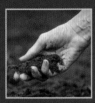

Soil Care & Fertility
Fertilizers
Soil Amendments
Soil Testing
Mycorrhizal Fungi

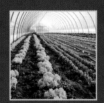

Weed & Disease Controls
Bactericides
Biological Fungicides
Cleaning & Sanitizing
Natural Herbicides

CALL TODAY!
1-800-827-2847
www.arbico-organics.com
CALL FOR FREE CATALOG

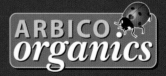

ARBICO
organics

*Providing Organic Solutions
For Growers Since 1979.*

01/2018

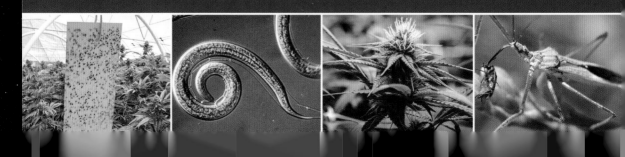

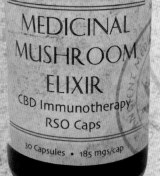
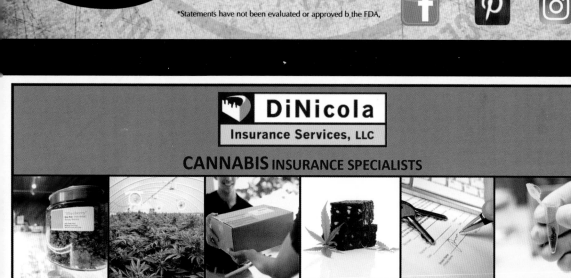
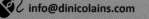

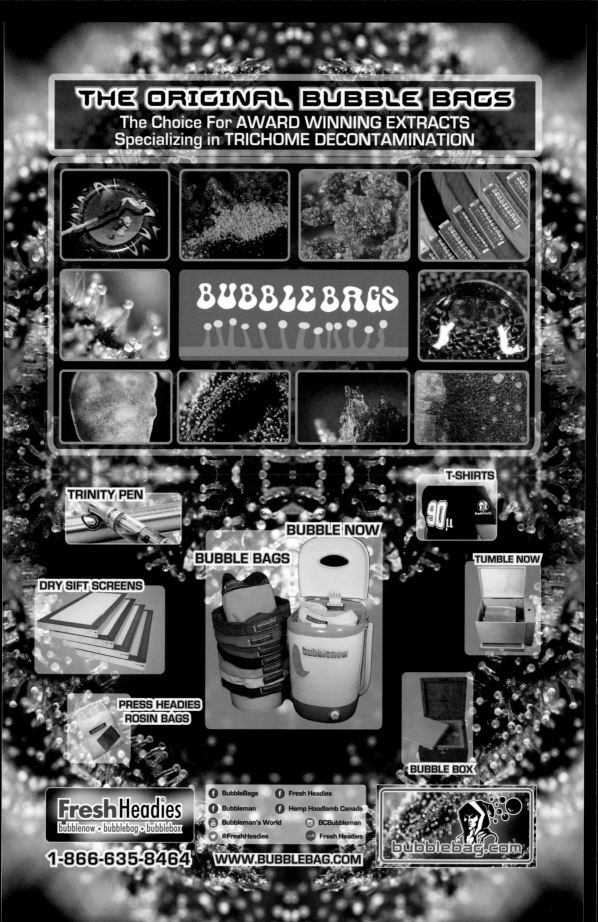

SEE, TASTE AND FEEL THE BOVEDA DIFFERENCE

EXPERIENCE 15% MORE TRICHOMES, CANNABINOIDS AND TERPENES

Boveda is made up of 100% natural water and salts. Based on the natural process of osmosis, Boveda releases and absorbs pure water to maintain the optimal humidity level for cannabis and creates a 100% stable and safe environment for curing and storing it.

Experience it yourself.

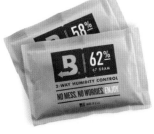

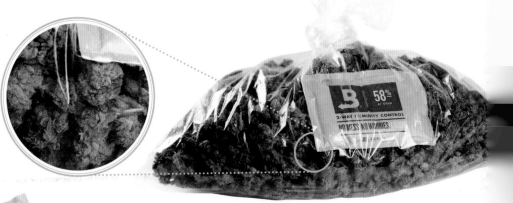

WITH BOVEDA

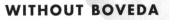

WITHOUT BOVEDA

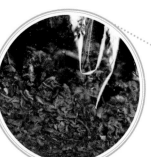

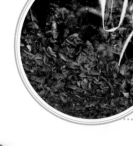

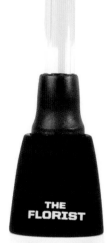